MAKING COGNITIVE-BEHAVIORAL THERAPY WORK

MAKING COGNITIVE-BEHAVIORAL THERAPY WORK

■ ■ ■

Clinical Process for New Practitioners

DEBORAH ROTH LEDLEY
BRIAN P. MARX
RICHARD G. HEIMBERG

THE GUILFORD PRESS
New York   London

© 2005 The Guilford Press
A Division of Guilford Publications, Inc.
72 Spring Street, New York, NY 10012
www.guilford.com

Printed in the United States of America

This book is printed on acid-free paper.

Last digit is print number: 9 8 7 6 5 4 3

Library of Congress Cataloging-in-Publication Data

Ledley, Deborah Roth.
  Making cognitive-behavioral therapy work : clinical process for new practitioners /
Deborah Roth Ledley, Brian P. Marx, Richard G. Heimberg.
    p. cm.
  Includes bibliographical references and index.
  ISBN 1-59385-142-1 (hardcover : alk. paper)
  1. Cognitive therapy. I. Marx, Brian P. II. Heimberg, Richard G. III. Title.
  RC489.C63L44 2005
  616.89'142—dc22

                                                                    2005001915

To my grandparents, Henry and Esther Bernick,
for giving me the gift of education and a love of learning

To my parents, Frank and Roslyn Roth,
for being the most loving and supportive
parents a person could wish for

And to Gary, the light of my life
—D. R. L.

For Denise and Colin, whom I love very much
—B. P. M.

To Poppi, who always makes me smile
To Tips, who always makes me feel appreciated
To Chris and Amy, who always make me proud
And most of all, to Linda, who lights up my life
—R. G. H.

ABOUT THE AUTHORS

Deborah Roth Ledley, PhD, was Assistant Professor of Psychology in Psychiatry at the University of Pennsylvania School of Medicine, as well as a faculty member at the Center for the Treatment and Study of Anxiety, from 2001 to 2005. She is currently in private practice in the Philadelphia area. Dr. Ledley's scholarly publications include articles and book chapters on the nature and treatment of social phobia, obsessive–compulsive disorder, and other anxiety disorders. She is also coeditor of *Improving Outcomes and Preventing Relapse in Cognitive-Behavioral Therapy.*

Brian P. Marx, PhD, is Associate Professor of Psychology at Temple University. Dr. Marx has written extensively about understanding, predicting, and controlling the sequelae to psychological trauma. He has also written about therapeutic processes that are important for behavior change.

Richard G. Heimberg, PhD, is Professor of Psychology, Director of Clinical Training, and Director of the Adult Anxiety Clinic of Temple University. He is also past president of the Association for Advancement of Behavior Therapy. Dr. Heimberg is well known for his efforts to develop and evaluate cognitive-behavioral treatments for social anxiety, and has published more than 250 articles and chapters on social anxiety, the anxiety disorders, and related topics. He is coeditor or coauthor of several books, including *Social Phobia: Diagnosis, Assessment, and Treatment; Managing Social Anxiety: A Cognitive-Behavioral Therapy Approach; Generalized Anxiety Disorder: Advances in Research and Practice;* and *Improving Outcomes and Preventing Relapse in Cognitive-Behavioral Therapy.*

ACKNOWLEDGMENTS

Early on in the preparation of this book, we formed an informal "advisory panel" of relatively new cognitive-behavioral therapists, some of whom were just beginning to see their first clients, and some of whom had completed their PhDs quite recently. The common concerns impacting beginning clinicians were fresh in the minds of everyone on our panel. We would like to thank Colleen Carney, Winnie Eng, Niki Jurburgs, Laura Lajos, Randi McCabe, Jennifer Mills, Karen Rowa, and Erin Scott for sharing their insights and helping to shape the content of the book. We would also like to thank all of the other students whom we have supervised over the years; each supervisory relationship highlights ways to better train students to be excellent cognitive-behavioral therapists. Finally, we would like to thank the excellent supervisors we have had, who not only started us on the path to being good therapists, but also imparted to us a model for delivering good training and supervision to others.

CONTENTS

Chapter 1   **Introducing Cognitive-Behavioral Process**   1
How to Gain Confidence as a Clinician   1
Preparing to See Clients   6
Cognitive-Behavioral Integration: Moving Beyond
      the "Black Box"   12

Chapter 2   **Initial Interactions with Clients**   20
The Initial Contact   20
Before Meeting the Client   23
In the Waiting Room   25
In the Room with the Client   25
The Case Conceptualization (Thus Far)   30
A Case Example   31

Chapter 3   **The Process of Assessment**   36
Being Mindful of Your Reactions   36
The Goals of Assessment   38
Tools for Accomplishing Assessment Goals   38
Common Concerns of Beginning Clinicians   54
Michael's Assessment Interview   56

Chapter 4   **Conceptualizing the Case and Planning Treatment**   62
Conceptualizing the Case   62
How Does the Case Conceptualization Inform
      the Treatment Plan?   71
Two Final Points on Treatment Planning   73

Chapter 5   **Giving Feedback to Clients and Writing the Assessment Report**   79
Reviewing the Client's Strengths   79
Reviewing the Problem List and Diagnoses   80
Sharing the Case Conceptualization   81

Reviewing Treatment Options 82
Michael's Feedback Session 85
Addressing Commonly Asked Questions about CBT 91
Writing the Report 97

Chapter 6   Starting the Cognitive-Behavioral Treatment Process   104
The Importance of Setting an Agenda 105
The First Treatment Session 106
Revisiting the Case of Michael 113
Before Moving On: A Note on Homework in CBT 128

Chapter 7   Dealing with Initial Challenges   130
in Cognitive-Behavioral Therapy
Challenges in Socializing Clients to CBT 130
Special Considerations for Clients Taking Medication
    While Doing CBT 134
Special Challenges: Working with Suicidal Clients 137
What Skills and Knowledge Do You Need to Assess
    Suicide Risk? 138
Clinician-Related Roadblocks That Can Interfere
    with Treatment 143
Difficult Interpersonal Situations in the
    Therapeutic Relationship 146

Chapter 8   The Next Sessions: Teaching the Core Techniques   154
Session 3: Introducing Cognitive Restructuring 155
Session 4: Continuing Cognitive Restructuring
    and Planning the First Exposure 160
Session 5: Doing the First Exposure 161
Sessions 6–10: Continuing Cognitive Restructuring
    and Exposures to Feared Situations 163
Keeping Good Client Records 165

Chapter 9   Managing Client Noncompliance   170
in Cognitive-Behavioral Therapy
Roadblock 1: Difficulties with Getting the Client
    to Engage in the Process of CBT 171
Roadblock 2: Client Difficulties with the
    Therapeutic Relationship 184
A Conclusion: Staying Positive in the Face
    of Challenges 195

Chapter 10   Terminating Therapy   196
Keeping the End Point in Mind 196
Teaching Clients to Be Their Own Clinicians 197
Things to Do in the Last Few Sessions of Therapy 201
Terminating Therapy: Staying the Course or
    Making Adjustments? 206
A Return to the Case of Michael 210

Contents

Chapter 11   **The Process of Supervision**   216
    The Goals of Supervision   216
    The Roles of the Supervisor   217
    The Role of the Trainee   218
    Setting Up a Supervisory Relationship   219
    Methods of Supervision   221
    Roadblocks in the Supervisory Relationship   224
    Focusing on the Positive   232

Appendix A   **Recommended Readings in Cognitive-Behavioral Therapy**   233

Appendix B   **Suggested Journals and Websites**   241

               References   243

               Index   247

MAKING COGNITIVE-BEHAVIORAL THERAPY WORK

Chapter 1

■ ■ ■

INTRODUCING COGNITIVE-BEHAVIORAL PROCESS

HOW TO GAIN CONFIDENCE AS A CLINICIAN

Every professional must do things for a first time. Architects must build their first building, teachers must teach their first class, surgeons must perform their first surgery. Similarly, beginning cognitive-behavioral clinicians must see their first clients. Learning new skills and beginning to develop in one's chosen profession can be very exciting, but these experiences can also be anxiety-provoking. One reason is that much of our work is unpredictable. At the beginning of a course of therapy, it is impossible to know whether or not clients will benefit. Many factors contribute to the outcome of therapy, and we are not able to manipulate all of these factors in a way that will guarantee a positive outcome. There are ways, however, to contend with this uncertainty.

The main goal of this book is to help beginning clinicians develop a sense of greater confidence and control as they start to work with clients. Throughout, we offer four main ways in which to gain this greater sense of confidence and control: engaging in preparation, understanding the process of cognitive-behavioral therapy (CBT), being mindful of possible difficulties, and making good use of supervision.

Preparation

The first thing that beginning clinicians can do in order to feel more confident about work with clients is to engage in adequate preparation. In some sense, "adequate preparation" is defined by one's training program, where specific requirements must be completed before trainees in-

1

teract with clients. However, training programs vary greatly in their requirements: Some allow trainees to begin working with clients shortly
after their arrival in the program and some require more extensive
coursework and clinical training before doing so. Logistical issues sometimes preclude what trainees may consider the ideal amount of preparation. For example, trainees might start to work with clients before having taken an ethics class simply because the course is scheduled later in
the curriculum. Finally, some trainees may seek out clinical experiences
for which their training program has not prepared them. For example,
someone who is in a psychodynamically focused training program might
decide that he or she would like to pursue training in CBT. This individual will begin seeing clients without the theoretical background to which
others are exposed in CBT-oriented programs. With these concerns in
mind, the section "Preparing to Conduct CBT" in this chapter offers beginning CBT clinicians additional suggestions that go beyond coursework, such as observing assessment and therapy sessions, reading very
widely in the field of CBT, and seeking out experiences (like national
conferences) in which you will be immersed in the cognitive-behavioral
way of conceptualizing and treating psychological problems.

Understanding the CBT Process and How to Make It Work

The whole process of therapy might seem elusive to beginning clinicians.
What must be accomplished over the course of therapy? What sort of
timeline should be followed? How can we ensure that our work with clients will progress in an organized manner?

We try to do away with some of this uncertainty by charting the
process of therapy from start to finish. Specifically, our work with clients
typically follows a standard progression of events: (1) orienting the client to the process of assessment and treatment, (2) performing an assessment and defining the problem(s) that will be the focus of treatment, (3)
creating a plan for treatment, (4) implementing the treatment program,
and (5) terminating treatment when appropriate. Throughout the book
this entire process is described, with a focus not only on how to accomplish necessary goals, but also how to deal with difficulties that can arise
at each stage.

Considered separately, each of the preceding five steps might seem
daunting, yet as CBT clinicians we are fortunate to have an overarching
theoretical framework that provides a way to understand and treat psychological difficulties. The cognitive-behavioral approach, as its name
implies, focuses on how problematic beliefs and behaviors play a role in
the development of psychological difficulties and, more importantly, in
the maintenance of these difficulties over time. Treatment entails chang-

ing these problematic beliefs and behaviors. Models for understanding specific disorders and difficulties have been advanced by cognitive-behavioral researchers and clinicians, and these models provide a road map for the process of therapy. (Useful resources for beginning clinicians are included in Appendix A.) They help the clinician and client to understand how various symptoms fit together and, working from that, to elucidate what changes need to be made in the service of symptom reduction. CBT does not progress blindly through treatment. Becoming familiar with these CBT models and using them as a framework for assessment and treatment will make you feel more comfortable with the process of therapy. Furthermore, educating your clients about these models will help them gain a coherent understanding of their own problems and how to go about resolving them.

Throughout the book, we also discuss how to make the CBT process work for you and your clients. There are two key process skills that help therapy progress effectively. They are establishing and maintaining a strong alliance with the individuals with whom we work and continuously working to understand our clients' difficulties and how to treat them. The latter skill is also called "case conceptualization." Both of these skill sets are briefly introduced here. Lessons on how to become skilled at both are integrated throughout this book.

Establishing and Maintaining the Therapeutic Alliance

The process of CBT involves a collaboration between clinician and client, which is facilitated by the development of a strong therapeutic alliance. Across diverse therapy approaches, a significant relationship has been found between quality of the therapeutic relationship and treatment outcome (Lambert & Bergin, 1994). In CBT, the therapeutic relationship is viewed as one between equals with differing areas of expertise. Whereas clinicians are trained to be experts in understanding and treating psychological problems, clients are viewed as "experts" in the particular difficulties that they are experiencing. The clients themselves are not "sick" or "abnormal"; rather, their problems make a great deal of sense within the context of learned dysfunctional beliefs and behaviors. CBT offers hope because it shows how such beliefs and behaviors can be "unlearned," and how more effective ways of thinking and behaving can be learned.

As assessment and treatment progress, it is the clinician's job to develop a clear understanding of clients' difficulties. This is only feasible, however, if both parties are willing to work together. Therefore, it is imperative that the clinician include the client in the therapy process as much as possible. The clinician's job is to develop a plan for treatment and to implement it, but the client should be involved each step of the way, providing the clinician with accurate information, working closely with him or her to develop a plan of action, following through with the implementation of this plan, and suggesting modifications where appropriate. As treatment progresses, the client should gradually be given more and more responsibility for implementing the plan. The goal of successful therapy is to teach clients the skills they need to become their own therapists. A strong, collaborative therapeutic alliance is essential to this goal.

Unfortunately, there is no set of rules or guidelines for establishing a good therapeutic relationship. However, we find it very helpful to draw on the work of Carl Rogers (1957), who emphasized empathy (the ability to see clients' worlds from their point of view), genuineness (allowing what we say and how we behave to be congruent with what we think and feel), and nonpossessive warmth (caring for clients, treating them with respect) as essential clinician qualities. He also encouraged a stance of unconditional positive regard, in which clients are accepted and valued for who they are. This idea of unconditional positive regard fits well with the stance of CBT clinicians, who typically do not blame clients for their symptoms. Symptoms are thought to be maintained via cognitive and behavioral pathways, not by laziness, lack of motivation, or weakness. Taken together, these Rogerian qualities have been found quite reliably to predict good treatment outcome in many forms of therapy, including CBT (see review by Keijsers, Schaap, & Hoogduin, 2000).

Although acting in a empathic, warm, and genuine way might not sound terribly difficult, these skills can easily be lost when our minds are on other things. Beginning clinicians may become excessively self-focused, worrying about the way that they are coming across to clients (e.g., "Do I look old enough?" or "Do I seem experienced enough?" and so forth) or about getting a job done correctly and efficiently (e.g., an assessment). This excessive self-focus may prevent clinicians from being themselves and from exhibiting the qualities that they inherently possess. To ameliorate this problem, beginning clinicians should make every effort to focus their attention on the client. Pay attention to what the client is saying and how the client is reacting to what you are saying. As you focus attention on the client and his or her difficulties, it is likely that he or she will feel more comfortable, supported, and understood.

Case Conceptualization

Case conceptualization is basically a working hypothesis of how the client's particular problems can be understood in terms of the cognitive-behavioral model. It is one of the most important skills that any clinician will learn. As with building and maintaining rapport, case conceptualization is a skill that is used over the entire process of assessment and treatment with every client. When we first meet clients, they tell us about difficult emotions, problematic behaviors, and troubling thoughts. They also provide important information about their family histories, stressful and traumatic life events, and the current state of their affairs. They might share with us past efforts at treatment, telling us about what did and did not work.

As a beginning clinician, all of this information might seem overwhelming and difficult to organize. However, cognitive-behavioral theory helps us to organize information, to develop hypotheses regarding the factors that maintain the client's current psychological difficulties, and to devise a plan for treatment. In other words, rather than seeing the client solely as a collection of symptoms, the process of conceptualization helps the clinician to think clearly about the reasons for, and the relationships among, these symptoms. In doing so, the apparent complexity of the client's emotional and behavioral difficulties is reduced to a manageable level. In Chapters 3–5, we discuss how to collect and organize the information you obtain in a meaningful way and to develop useful hypotheses about your client based on this information. The process of case conceptualization is much like putting together a jigsaw puzzle— the parts must fit together in a logical fashion. Clinicians must develop a coherent understanding of the difficulties that clients are having as well as a plan for how to help clients resolve these difficulties. Furthermore, even after the development of the initial conceptualization and treatment plan, case conceptualization remains an essential ingredient of successful therapy. As we discuss throughout this book, both assessment and case conceptualization are ongoing processes because our understanding of the nature of a client's psychological problems will likely change as we acquire new information from session to session.

As in all aspects of CBT, the case conceptualization should be a collaborative process. Following a baseline assessment, the case conceptualization should be shared with the client. The way in which it is shared is critical. Rather than dictating to the client how the clinician has come to understand the case, the clinician should present it as a hypothesis and provide the client with the opportunity to make adjustments. This should occur throughout treatment.

Being Mindful of Potential Difficulties

It is a great help to know in advance the kinds of difficulties that can arise over the course of CBT. In the ideal world, establishing a strong therapeutic relationship would be easy, clients would always comply with treatment, and they would always make the kinds of changes that their clinicians would like them to make. In the real world, therapy rarely progresses that smoothly. Although challenges can make our work stressful, they also keep it stimulating and vital.

It is very difficult to predict when challenges will arise in CBT and what form they will take. However, beginning clinicians can benefit greatly from knowing what kind of challenges can arise and various ways in which they can be handled. Throughout the book, but especially in Chapters 7 and 9, we shed light on just these issues.

Making Good Use of Supervision

Beginning clinicians can ease some of the anxiety they experience by making good use of supervision. This topic is covered in Chapter 11, the final chapter of the book. Beginning clinicians might *feel* alone when they start to see clients, but in fact, they are not. Rather, trainees have the benefit of being supervised by more experienced clinicians who can share with them their collective experiences from working with numerous clients over the course of their careers. In Chapter 11 we describe how to get the most out of supervision and how to deal with difficulties that may arise in the supervisory relationship.

Being a clinician is an exciting career choice. Most of us embark on this path because we want to help people. The process of doing so is never boring. Each client we see is unique, both in terms of his or her presentation and in terms of the alliance that is formed with the clinician. Even clients who progress through treatment quite uneventfully present interesting challenges to think through. Starting out as a clinician can indeed be stressful, but we encourage you to embark upon this path with a spirit of curiosity.

In the rest of this chapter, we offer suggestions for how to prepare for assessment and therapy.

PREPARING TO SEE CLIENTS

Beginning clinicians frequently seek advice on how best to prepare to see clients. Seeking this sort of information is an excellent anxiety-reduction technique. Having a sense of what may occur when we walk into a room with a client most certainly increases our confidence. Furthermore, when we are less focused on our own anxiety, we can better provide care to our clients.

One caveat deserves mention before we proceed. Some beginning clinicians put off seeing their first clients because they do not yet feel sufficiently prepared. While it is certainly appropriate to read about clinical activities, observe other people doing therapy or assessment, and practice these activities in role plays, the best way to learn how to assess and treat clients is to actually engage in these activities. In short, more practice makes us more skillful. This chapter offers some tips on how to build a good framework of knowledge and skill that will underlie the hands-on clinical work that will soon follow.

Getting Emotionally Prepared

Typically, beginning clinicians are plagued by insecurities about their abilities. Learning to reduce some of this anxiety requires an examination of what drives it. One source of difficulty is often unrealistic expectations of what it means to be competent in the provision of clinical services. Novices often fear they will be incompetent. Even though our skills as clinicians can only develop through experience, it is unrealistic for novices to expect complete failure simply because they are novices. In fact, research examining the relationship between clinician experience and therapy outcome is surprisingly inconsistent. Some studies have found a positive correlation between experience and outcome (e.g., Crits-Christoph et al., 1991; Smith & Glass, 1977), but in general these correlations have been modest. Other studies have found clinician experience to be unrelated to treatment outcome (e.g., Shapiro & Shapiro, 1982) and to therapy dropout rates (Wierzbicki & Pekarik, 1993).

In light of these findings, beginning clinicians should not hold fast to the belief that their lack of experience will negatively affect their clients. Most individuals who choose to embark on a career as clinicians possess skills that have made them and others believe that this choice was suited to them. It is likely that these skills match those described by Rogers—empathy, genuineness, and nonpossessive warmth. When combined with good preparation (as described in the remainder of this chapter) and strong supervision (as discussed in Chapter 11), it is likely that even beginning clinicians will confer some benefits on their clients.

Another problem that can sap the confidence of beginning clinicians is an unrealistic definition of successful outcome in therapy. Many beginning clinicians believe that successful therapy is defined as the removal of all symptoms and problems within a specified (typically brief) period of time. Not only is this belief unfair to the clinician, it is also unfair to the client. In many cases, clients do not improve as much as we might hope. Thus, the goal of completely resolving every client problem is unrealistic and can set beginning clinicians up for failure. It is more reasonable to tell yourself "My goal is to orient the client to cognitive-behavioral approaches to understanding and treating a particular problem. I will teach my client those cognitive and behavioral techniques that have been shown to be effective for treating that problem." This goal is reasonable, easy to measure, and not particularly dependent on many client variables over which you may have little influence.

Understanding the Theory Behind CBT

It is beyond the scope of this book to cover the theory behind CBT in any depth. However, we try here to briefly give some insight into its theoretical underpinnings. Through both coursework and further reading (see our recommendations in Appendix A), beginning cognitive-behavioral clinicians should develop a strong knowledge base in the theory underlying the work that we do with clients.

CBT is currently an integration of two originally separate theoretical approaches to understanding and treating psychological disorders: the behavioral approach and the cognitive approach. The behavioral approach (at its strictest) focuses exclusively on observable, measurable behavior and ignores all mental events. It views the mind/brain as a "black box" not worthy of exploration. It focuses instead on the interactions of environment and behavior. The cognitive approach focuses on the role of mind, and specifically on cognitions as determinants of feelings and behaviors.

The Behavioral Approach

John B. Watson, often considered to be the "father of behaviorism," saw all behavior, and all behavior change, as a function of learning via *classical conditioning*. He posited that even complex behaviors could be broken down into component behaviors that had all been acquired through simple learning processes. There are three key elements of classical conditioning: (1) the unconditioned stimulus and response, (2) the conditioned stimulus, and (3) the conditioned response. The unconditioned stimulus is any stimulus that is capable of producing a particular reflexive response. An example of an unconditioned stimulus is food—it naturally elicits salivation, an unconditioned response. The conditioned stimulus is one that is neutral prior to being paired with an unconditioned stimulus. For example, if a baby is shown a green light, he would have no particular response to it (beyond looking at it). But if the baby was repeatedly presented with the green light immediately before his mother began to feed him, he would eventually start to salivate in response to the green light alone. Salivation has now become a conditioned response—with repeated pairings, the conditioned stimulus (the green light) now elicits the same response (salivation) that occurred with the unconditioned stimulus alone (food). Watson believed that all learning (and thus, all behavior change) occurs through this type of simple stimulus–response pairings.

Here are some more examples that clearly show classical conditioning at work in the kinds of problematic behavior that CBT therapists are interested in. Watson and his colleague, Rosalie Rayner, did a famous experiment with a little boy named Albert. Albert had never seen a rat, and thus had no learned response to it. In other words, the white rat was a "neutral stimulus" for Albert. Watson and Rayner showed Albert the rat, at the same time pairing it with a loud noise (unconditioned stimulus). The noise was known to elicit a startle or fear response (unconditioned response) in Albert. Within just seven pairings of the white rat and the loud noise, Albert came to exhibit a fear response (conditioned response) to the rat alone (conditioned stimulus). Albert had "learned" to fear the rat. In fact, Albert came to fear many white, furry objects, including rabbits and a mask of Santa Claus. In behavioral terms, Albert's fear "generalized" to other white, furry objects. Another study, referred to as the case of Little Peter (Jones, 1924) demonstrated how fears could also be "unlearned." A young boy named Peter who was afraid of rabbits (the origin of his fear was not known) was exposed to a rabbit in a cage while eating lunch for many days. Peter came to no longer fear the rabbit, leading the experimenters to assume that Peter developed a new association between rabbits and the pleasure of eating lunch, rather than between rabbits and fear. These early experiments in learning and "unlearning" are important to our current understanding of how people acquire fears and how we can then help to extinguish these fears.

B. F. Skinner was another key figure in the rise of behaviorism. Skinner's theories of conditioning were more sophisticated than Watson's; they focused on *operant* rather than classical conditioning. In operant conditioning, stimuli are not thought of as eliciting responses. Instead, as organisms interact with their environments, they emit all sorts of responses (called operants); when the organism is rewarded for a particular response, the response is more likely to occur again; in behavioral terms it has been "reinforced." Let's look at an example of operant conditioning at work in the kinds of problem we see as clinicians. Consider a child who cries before school and is then permitted to stay home from school by his mother. He greatly enjoys his day at home, spending time with his mom (whom he usually has to share with his siblings), watching TV, and playing video games. This child is likely to continue crying each morning since he has learned that this behavior yields a desired consequence. If the mother then reads in a parenting magazine that she should make her child go to school regardless of his crying, the crying behavior will eventually be extinguished since the child will learn that crying no longer yields the desired outcome. In other words, he will "unlearn" the association between crying and staying home from school.

The purely behavioral approach does apply to the some of the problems that we see as cognitive-behavioral therapists. However, simple stimulus–response associations cannot explain all learned behaviors. As the complexity of the behavioral phenomena increase, we require more complex explanations for behaviors. Knowing what people are thinking and feeling is also very important to understanding their behavior.

The Cognitive Approach

The cognitive approach most clearly deviates from the strictly behavioral approach when contrasted to the staunch behaviorists' "black box" view of the mind. The cognitive model is interested in the mind. Specifically, thoughts are considered important because they serve as the intervening variable between stimuli and our responses to them.

The cognitive model, and the therapy associated with it, is most closely associated with Aaron T. Beck. Beck developed cognitive therapy in the early 1960s as a treatment for depression, but it has since been applied to virtually every psychiatric disorder, as well as to general "problems of daily living." Cognitive therapy is based on the cognitive model, which proposes that distorted or dysfunctional thinking underlies all psychological disturbances. Furthermore, dysfunctional thinking has an important effect on our mood and behavior. The key concept of the cognitive model is that *it is not events themselves that affect our behavior, but rather how we perceive events.*

Let's use an example to illustrate this key concept. Consider this situation: Jane makes plans to meet a friend for a movie at 7 P.M. It is now 7:30; Jane's friend has not arrived and the movie is about to begin. What is Jane's response to this event? Jane, a chronic worrier, immediately assumes that her friend has been in a car accident on the way to the movies. This makes Jane feel terribly worried and anxious. Jane tries calling her friend's cell phone, but no one answers. She has vivid images of her friend in a totaled car in the middle of the freeway. She keeps calling, thinking that if her friend is trapped in the car, but conscious, she might answer and Jane would be able to offer her support. So Jane stands outside the movies, calling her friend repeatedly, and becoming increasingly panicked about her friend's fate and her inability to help her.

Another person might have a very different reaction. John might think that his friend decided she does not like doing things with him and has made plans to see another friend instead. This might make John feel dejected, and might lead him to go home and have a good cry. Susan might think that her friend just forgot to meet her, as she has often done in the past. This might leave Susan feeling annoyed, and she might then decide to head into the movies on her own. Jeff might think that maybe *he* got the time or date wrong. This would leave him feeling rather careless, and he might head to the store on his way home to buy the appointment book that he has been meaning to get for weeks. This example illustrates that a single situation can elicit various emotional and behavioral responses, all depending on how the person *perceives* the situation. This is really the crux of the cognitive model.

The cognitive model, as set forth by Beck (and illustrated in Figure 1.1), begins with central core beliefs. These beliefs about oneself, other people, and the world form during childhood based on the experiences that we have as we are growing up. Core beliefs are "understandings that are so fundamental and deep that they . . . are regarded by the person as absolute truths, just the way things 'are' " (J. S. Beck, 1995, p. 15). Core beliefs are global and apply to situations in general. This is in contrast to automatic thoughts, which are described as "the actual words or images that go through a person's mind" and which are situation-specific. In between core beliefs and automatic thoughts are intermediary beliefs, which consist of "attitudes, rules and assumptions" (J. S. Beck, 1995, p. 16). Let's return to our example of Jane to illustrate

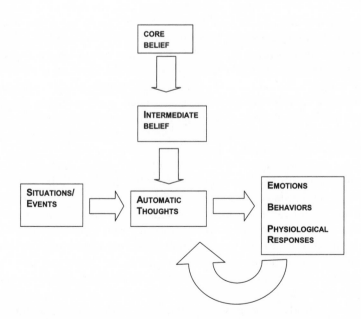

FIGURE 1.1. The cognitive model. Adapted from J. S. Beck (1995, p. 18). Copyright 1995 by The Guilford Press. Adapted by permission.

these concepts. It is certainly possible that Jane holds a core belief that "I'm an unlucky person." In between this core belief and her automatic thought ("My friend was in an accident"), Jane might hold a variety of intermediate beliefs, including "Bad things will happen to people I am close to" and "The world is full of danger."

The cognitive model posits that when people find themselves in situations, automatic thoughts are activated that are directly influenced by their core beliefs and intermediate beliefs. Automatic thoughts then influence our reactions. Because our most fundamental beliefs impact our thoughts in any given situation, different people have very different reactions to the same situations.

COGNITIVE-BEHAVIORAL INTEGRATION: MOVING BEYOND THE "BLACK BOX"

In the cognitive model, stimuli consist of an event plus our interpretation of (our thoughts about) the event. Stimuli may also consist of thoughts by themselves. When referring to responses or "reactions," the cognitive model is referring to three kinds of reactions: emotional, behavioral, and physiological. When Jane automatically concludes that her friend has been in a car crash on the way to the movies, she feels worried (emoion), calls her friend repeatedly on the cell phone to see if she is okay (behavior), and experiences all sorts of physical symptoms like shaking, sweating, and shortness of breath. All of these reactions are a result of the way Jane interpreted a situation that could have been interpreted (and therefore reacted to) in a number of different ways. As is illustrated in Figure 1.1, these reactions then feed back into automatic thoughts. For example, when Jane's friend did not answer after a few calls, Jane's next automatic thought was "She must be dead." Her friend's non-response served to confirm Jane's beliefs.

So, how does CBT work? We will discuss the workings of CBT throughout this book, but on the most basic level, techniques that fall under the umbrella of CBT work to change parts of this chain of events from situation to interpretation to reaction. As illustrated in Figure 1.2, CBT involves both cognitive and behavioral treatment tools. It would be overly simplistic though to think that cognitive techniques only target cognitions and behavioral techniques only target behaviors. As Figure 1.2 shows, change in one of these systems undoubtedly results in change in the other systems.

Let's consider first how this applies with cognitive techniques. Our primary cognitive tool is cognitive restructuring, which involves identifying and reframing maladaptive thoughts. Rather than treating automatic

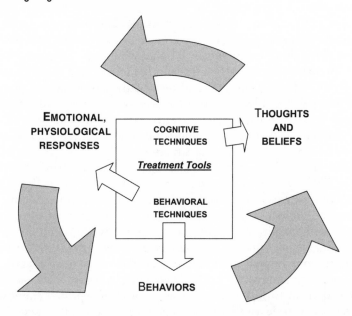

FIGURE 1.2. Basic model for cognitive-behavioral case conceptualization.

thoughts as "truths," cognitive restructuring involves questioning our thoughts and reframing them if they are irrational or maladaptive. Let's return to Jane, but imagine that this same scenario plays out when Jane is just starting cognitive therapy. Jane's automatic response to her friend being late is still to assume that her friend has been in a terrible accident and died. However, given her newfound CBT skills, she is now able to question these thoughts. She quite quickly realizes that she has jumped to conclusions, that there are all sorts of possible reasons for why her friend is late, and that it is unlikely that her friend is dead. Jane recognizes that her friend might be running late, might have gotten lost, might have had something come up at work, and might have also forgotten to turn her cell phone on. These realizations lead to a very different behavioral response. Jane decides to leave a message on her friend's cell phone saying she is going to go in and see the movie, and telling her friend to either come in and meet her if she is running late or call back later to let her know what happened. This is very different behaviorally than standing outside the movie theater, calling her friend repeatedly in a panic. Jane is also likely to have different emotional and physiological reactions. As she settles in to the theater and begins to enjoy the movie, she will likely feel calm and relaxed, rather than terribly anxious.

What did Jane learn from CBT? Her most important lesson was

that a single situation has many possible interpretations. She also learned that there are various ways to react to a single situation. She learned that calling her friend in a panic would not have been of any benefit (to her, or her friend!) and she learned that going to see the movie turned out to be pleasant and had no negative consequences (e.g., her fear of being unavailable to a friend in need was not realized). The act of cognitive restructuring positively affected Jane's beliefs (as we would expect), her behavioral responses, and her emotional and physiological responses to a potentially stressful situation.

How does this reciprocal relationship apply with behavioral techniques? There are many behavioral tools under the umbrella of CBT, such as *in vivo* exposure, social skills training, relaxation training, and structured problem solving. However, a commonality of all of these tools, as with cognitive restructuring, is that they are based in learning theory and involve unlearning old, maladaptive associations between stimuli and our responses while also learning new ones. *In vivo* exposure, for example, involves helping people to confront harmless stimuli that cause them to feel anxious. The purpose of repeated exposure to such triggers is to learn that their anxieties are unfounded. Take for example, Stan, a man with a terrible phobia of snakes. For as long as he could remember, Stan was terrified of all snake-related stimuli (e.g., pictures of snakes, snakes in movies). He recently purchased a house, and relished the idea of gardening. But he soon learned that his garden contained small garden-variety snakes. The few times that he saw one, he had terribly frightening thoughts (e.g., "It's going to bite me," "I'm going to die from its venom," "I can't cope with this"). These thoughts led him to feel very anxious (emotional reaction) and experience racing heart and sweating (physiological responses). Each time he saw one of these tiny snakes in his garden, he ran away and would not come outside for days afterward until someone could come over to his house and confirm that the snake was no longer in the garden (behavioral response). His garden soon became overgrown from neglect, and the neighbors were starting to complain.

Stan decided to get some treatment, and chose to see a behavior therapist. Treatment involved repeated exposure first to snake-related stimuli, and gradually to real snakes. With repeated exposure, Stan gradually came to exhibit a neutral response to snakes and, later, actually came to like snakes so much that he not only returned to gardening, but also bought a snake as a pet. Rather than associating the snake with fear and terror, he came to associate it with pleasure and liking.

It seems as if Stan's treatment was purely behavioral—with repeated exposure, he set up a new stimulus–response association. Yet how did this new association become established? It certainly seems that Stan developed some new *beliefs* about snakes. As he learned more about them through exposure, he learned that most snakes where he lived do not bite and are not poisonous. He learned that snakes are not slimy feeling (as he predicted before his first exposure), but that they are actually dry, smooth and quite nice to touch. And, he also learned that it could be enjoyable and interesting to watch snakes move through various habitats and engage in their natural behaviors like eating and burrowing under the sand. These learning experiences led to an extinction of one stimulus-response pairing (snakes-fear) and the formation of a new stimulus-response pairing (snakes-pleasure). This new association led to a shift in beliefs ("I like snakes," "Snakes aren't scary") and a shift in behavior (e.g., gardening, buying a snake as a pet, etc.), even though treatment—on the surface—appeared to be focused simply on "behavior."

Preparing to Do Assessments

Before we begin to treat clients, it is essential to do a thorough evaluation. Assessment often has two goals. The first is to establish a diagnosis based on the *Diagnostic and Statistical Manual of Mental Disorders*, 4th edition, text revision (DSM-IV-TR; American Psychiatric Association, 2000). Not all clinical settings utilize the DSM diagnostic system, but many CBT settings do, and it is therefore important to learn it well. The other goal of assessments is universal—to form a conceptualization, or theoretical understanding, of the case that will serve as a guide for treatment. In other words, CBT therapists seek to answer the following questions: What particular dysfunctional thoughts lead to the client's specific emotional and behavioral problems? How, then, does problematic emotion and behavior feed back into the maintenance of dysfunctional cognition?

Assessment for Diagnosis

How can a beginning clinician prepare to meet the first goal of assessment—that is, to establish diagnoses based on the DSM system? Although diagnostic skills are honed only through experience, clinicians must start doing assessments with a strong background in diagnostic classification. This means being very familiar with the diagnostic criteria for at least the most common of the psychological disorders. Although we do not need to memorize these criteria, we should know the general description of the various disorders and how to distinguish one disorder from another. Many disorders have common features and, as you speak to clients, you must ask appropriate questions to arrive at a differential diagnosis.

The best way to correctly arrive at a DSM diagnosis for a particular constellation of symptoms is to use a semistructured clinical interview designed just for this purpose (these are described in more detail in Chapter 3). It is essential that clinicians are familiar with such interviews before they begin to use them with clients. Appropriate preparation should involve getting a clear sense of what the interview is all about, learning how to phrase questions, becoming familiar with the rules for administration (e.g., providing clients with specific definitions of concepts, adhering to time limits, etc.) and knowing how to progress from one section of the interview to another. This knowledge can be acquired by reading manuals or watching training tapes, observing a colleague or supervisor conducting an assessment, and/or by conducting an assessment with a colleague or supervisor. In our view, one of the best ways to learn to do assessments is to watch an experienced clinician assess a few clients and then to conduct a few assessments with an experienced clinician watching you. Following each assessment, beginning clinicians should be given feedback and should also be afforded the opportunity to ask questions.

Watching experienced clinicians (either on training tapes or in person) can be intimidating at first. Interviews seem to flow gracefully from topic to topic, giving the observer the sense that the interviewer knows exactly what path should be followed to accurately complete the assessment. As we have already noted, these skills come both from preparation (becoming familiar with the interview format, knowing the diagnostic criteria) and from practice. With that being said, it is also essential that you hold reasonable expectations for yourself. At one time, these very skilled interviewers felt just as awkward as you feel now.

Assessment for Case Conceptualization

A DSM diagnosis tells you only one thing: whether the symptoms your client is experiencing fit together into a recognizable disorder or syndrome. Certainly, we have knowledge associated with many diagnostic entities—how prevalent they are, whether they are more common in women or in men, the mean age of onset, etc. Nevertheless, these "factual" data do not equal an *understanding* of the client. Being able to assign a name to a group of symptoms does not mean that you know how these symptoms started or what keeps them going. This is where CBT theory and case conceptualization come in. Clinicians need to know how to go beyond simple diagnosis and come to an understanding—within a CBT framework—of why a client has a particular problem. The clinician therefore will want to gather information on the client's specific thoughts about his or her problems, about emotional and behavioral responses, and about antecedents and consequences of those responses.

Like diagnostic skill, developing the ability to conceptualize cases comes with time and experience. Once you begin working with clients, you should share your ongoing conceptualizations of cases during your weekly supervision meetings. It can also be very beneficial to participate in a supervision group, where you can hear conceptualizations of other clinicians' cases and share your own. In such settings, it is important to be open to different ways of understanding cases. Remember that the case conceptualization is a work in progress that can be adjusted based on your insights into the client's problems, the client's own insights, and sometimes the considerations of other professionals as well.

There are also some excellent sources to read on case conceptualization. A must-read for all beginning clinicians is *Cognitive Therapy in Practice: A Case Formulation Approach* written by Jacqueline B. Persons (1989). We discuss Persons's approach in much greater detail in Chapter 4. Another good source for case conceptualization material is the second chapter of Judith S. Beck's (1995) *Cognitive Therapy: Basics and Beyond*.

Preparing to Conduct CBT

Once an assessment is complete, the case has been conceptualized and a treatment plan devised, the work of the clinician is only just beginning. How should a beginning clinician prepare to actually conduct CBT? One important component to preparation is reading. Having a good knowledge base about the range of techniques that fall under the CBT umbrella is essential. Perhaps the best resource available for elucidating the core techniques of CBT is Judith S. Beck's 1995 book, *Cognitive Therapy: Basics and Beyond*. Many beginning clinicians also find the following books helpful in learning these core techniques:

- *Feeling Good: The New Mood Therapy* by David Burns (1980).
- *Mind over Mood* by Dennis Greenberger and Christine Padesky (1995; see also Padesky and Greenberger's [1995] *Clinician's Guide to Mind Over Mood*).
- *Cognitive Therapy Techniques: A Practitioner's Guide* by Robert L. Leahy (2003).
- *Cognitive Therapy and the Emotional Disorders* by Aaron T. Beck (1976).
- *Cognitive Therapy of Depression* by Aaron T. Beck, A. John Rush, Brian F. Shaw, and Gary Emery (1979).

Once beginning clinicians have a handle on the core techniques of CBT, they must acquire knowledge about cognitive-behavioral theories and therapy for specific psychological problems. A good place to start is with a very broad book like the third edition of David H. Barlow's (2001) *Clinical Handbook of Psychological Disorders: A Step-by-Step Treatment Manual.* The book includes chapters on a number of specific psychological problems that outline the nature of each problem, cognitive-behavioral models for understanding them, and how to use CBT to treat them from initial assessment to termination. The book provides an excellent model of how CBT is applied to different psychological problems and an excellent blend of data (prevalence rates, findings from treatment outcome studies) and practical knowledge (case examples, sample dialogues, forms for clients to complete, etc.).

When you begin to treat clients with specific difficulties, more in-depth reading in specific areas is also important (see Appendix A for resources). This in-depth reading should include research-oriented books (e.g., books that discuss epidemiology, etiology, diagnostic issues, approaches to treatment, etc.), as well as treatment manuals. Some manuals include brief overviews of research on the specific problem, but are, of course, most specifically focused on guiding clinicians through the treatment process.

Unfortunately, simply reading books and treatment manuals will not allow you to keep up to date on cutting-edge knowledge in our field. Practicing clinicians should make a habit of keeping up to date on influential treatment outcome studies, as well as studies that help us to better understand the nature of various psychological disturbances. There are too many excellent journals in our field to list them all here, but we have included the names of some that beginning clinicians might want to start keeping up with in Appendix B.

In addition to reading, beginning clinicians can also prepare to conduct CBT by watching more experienced clinicians. It can be quite informative (and fun) to watch the "masters" of CBT on videotape. The Association for Advancement of Behavior Therapy has created a series called the "World Rounds Videotapes" that shows world-renowned cognitive-behavioral clinicians treating clients. These videos afford the opportunity to see excellent CBT, often from the individuals who created the treatments for specific problems.

Since the "World Rounds" series shows an abridged version of therapy, beginning clinicians should also try to secure videotapes of entire cases. Many training clinics maintain tapes of interesting cases for trainees to watch. By watching a case from start to finish, you will not only to be exposed to many different therapy techniques, but also to issues that can come up at different stages of the therapy process. Whenever possible, novice clinicians should discuss their observations with a more experienced clinician, ideally the clinician who did the treatment. In this way, you can ask the clinician to explain why he or she made the decisions that were made as the therapy progressed.

Therapy sessions can also be observed in real time from behind a one-way mirror or in the room with the clinician and client. This is an excellent way to learn, particularly if you can spend some time with the clinician after each session to discuss the case and ask questions. If you are able to be in the room with the clinician and client, you might also be able to take a gradually more active role, depending on the style of the clinician and the willingness of the client. These parameters should be discussed with the clinician, and also with the client, prior to the beginning of the case so that everyone is clear on the nature of your role.

The best way to really learn how to conduct CBT is to . . . conduct CBT. We discuss supervision in great detail in Chapter 11 of this book, outlining how best to make use of the supervisory relationship as you begin to treat clients of your own.

One Final Tip

As a beginning CBT clinician, it is also advisable to join international, national, or local organizations. Membership in these organizations allows you to keep informed about current developments in cognitive-behavioral research and practice. These organizations also sponsor conferences where you can learn by attending workshops and talks and where you can meet other individuals who are also interested in CBT. These organizations include the Association for the Advancement of Behavior Therapy and the International Association for Cognitive Psychotherapy, as well as more specialized organizations like the Anxiety Disorders Association of America. The Academy of Cognitive Therapy (ACT) is another excellent resource. The ACT offers certification to individuals with advanced expertise in cognitive therapy, but also offers resources pertinent to beginning clinicians, including listings of clinical psychology doctoral programs, internships, and postdoctoral fellowships that have a CBT focus.

Chapter 2

■　■　■

INITIAL INTERACTIONS WITH CLIENTS

Depending on the nature of your job and the environment in which you work, your initial contact with clients will vary. Some clinicians take phone calls from potential clients; some are assigned clients and their first contact involves calling to set up a first appointment; and some do not have contact with clients until they actually come in for their first visit.

In this chapter we will lead you through a hypothetical progression of events that is typical, even if it does not exactly match your specific clinical setting. By following this progression, however, we will be able to illustrate the process of becoming acquainted with clients. Most importantly, we will focus on establishing rapport with new clients, as well as using early interactions with clients to inform case conceptualization.

THE INITIAL CONTACT

Regardless of the nature of the client's initial contact, taking this first step in seeking help can be a daunting task for many people. We have all met clients who have considered calling for months, or even years, before actually doing so. Given these circumstances, it is important to be sensitive to the client's situation and any discomfort or awkwardness that he or she might be feeling. It is also important to keep in mind that an initial phone contact or visit is typically not the appropriate arena in which to thoroughly assess and diagnose a client's difficulties. Rather, it should be used as the context in which to obtain basic and relevant information in order to determine the next appropriate step.

A good starting place with any potential client is to ask for a brief description of the kinds of difficulties that he or she has been having. This can be accomplished by asking questions like "How can I help you today?" or "What is it that led you to call us today?" or "What sorts of difficulties have you been having recently?" Some individuals will quite easily and clearly answer the question, providing the clinician with an opportunity for further questions. Others might be reluctant to disclose information over the phone or talk in detail about their problems because of shame or embarrassment about their difficulties or the need to seek treatment. In these situations, it is essential that you communicate your willingness to help the individual and allow him or her as much time as needed to share information with you. It is only after you have adequate information that you will be able to make appropriate recommendations.

A good first step to getting past initial anxieties experienced by callers is to reinforce their "sharing" behavior by telling them that that you are glad that they called and that you know how hard it can be to share very personal and distressing information. Second, if appropriate, it can be very helpful to normalize people's concerns ("The difficulties that you are having are very similar to those experienced by many people who call our clinic") and to reassure them that you are available to help them. Once individuals do begin to talk, it is essential that you react to what they tell you in an understanding, calm, and nonjudgmental way. Once this tone is established, most clients will feel comfortable continuing to speak to you about their difficulties.

Making Recommendations

The clinician's goal for the initial conversation is to make a recommendation for how the individual should proceed. There are many options to consider. One possibility is to bring the person in for a more in-depth evaluation. Another option is to refer individuals to another professional or clinic if neither you nor any of your colleagues are able to treat them. This should be handled in a way that is sensitive to the possibility that the caller may feel rejected by such a suggestion. For example, he or she can be told, "It sounds like your main problems right now have to do with your marital relationship. We don't do couples therapy at our clinic, so let me give you some recommendations in the area where you can pursue that kind of treatment." It is always best to give callers a few options just in case a particular clinician is not taking new clients or does not take the kind of insurance that the person has. It is also good practice to invite the individual to call you back if none of the referrals work out.

Sometimes, individuals contact clinicians to gather information rather than to seek treatment. In some cases, they just are not ready to commit to therapy but are at the stage in which they want to learn more about their problems or attend a support group. Again, information should be provided, along with an invitation to call back should they want treatment in the future. At other times, we as clinicians might sense that treatment is not necessary. For instance, individuals might call and describe very minimal symptoms and might feel concerned about finding time to come in for treatment. In such cases, recommendations for self-help books, websites, or local support groups can be provided. These more minimal interventions can be sufficient for some people; others might give them a try and then see that it is worth making the sacrifices required for participation in more structured treatment. In general, when potential clients call a clinician, they want to come away with *something*— an appointment, a referral, or information. Leave them with the sense that calling to speak to a clinician was a positive decision, resulting in some positive changes.

Before moving on, it is important to emphasize that we should provide information to individuals during this initial contact slowly and in terms that are easy to understand. Avoid psychological jargon, keep information simple and straightforward, and make sure that you provide an opportunity for the individual to ask questions.

Making the Arrangements for a First Visit

Let us assume that the caller is a suitable candidate for assessment at the clinic in which you work. The next step, then, is setting up an initial visit. When inviting individuals to come in, clinicians should inform them of the purpose of the visit and what it will entail. Keeping in mind that anxiety can make it difficult for people to attend to details, make sure that they are clear on when the session will be held (date and time), how long the session will last, and, most importantly, how to get there. Some individuals will be so focused on making the initial phone call that they might forget to ask for these details and might then feel ashamed about needing to call back for further information. Be sure to provide all the necessary information and make sure that all of it is clear.

Asking Permission to Send an Advance Mailing

At the time a first session is arranged, an advance mailing can be sent reminding clients of the time of their appointment and providing them with directions for how to get there, contact information should they need to change their appointment, and perhaps some general information on the clinic or on the types of difficulties for which the individual is seeking help. It can also be very helpful to send questionnaires to clients and ask that they be completed before the assessment session. In this way, questionnaires can be used to facilitate the assessment process (see Chapter 3).

Before doing any of this, it is important to ask clients if it is okay to send mail to them. Some clients do not want family members to know that they are seeking treatment and might prefer that mail not be sent to their homes. When mailings are sent, unmarked envelopes should be used and marked confidential. At this point in your contact with clients, it is best to defer to their wishes on these issues. Be mindful, however, that these concerns can be important to the case conceptualization, and once therapy is underway, might become a focus of clinical attention. For example, a client who is very isolated and perceives that she lacks social support might benefit greatly from becoming more open with family members about the kinds of difficulties that she is having.

Setting the Fee

Prior to coming in for an assessment (and prior to beginning therapy as well), clients must be informed of how much the assessment will cost. In some settings, fee arrangements are handled by a business administrator and kept separate from the therapeutic relationship. In other settings, clinicians must take care of these arrangements themselves. Regardless of who deals with fee setting and collection, it is essential to note that the American Psychological Association's (APA) *Ethical Principles of Psychologists and Code of Conduct* (2002) requires that fees and financial arrangements be discussed "as early as is feasible" (code 6.04a). Beyond discussing your rates with clients, it is also important that you explain your policies on unpaid fees and missed appointments. Be knowledgeable about the policies at your clinic and be sure to explain these policies to clients clearly and in language that they can understand. Clients should sign a document agreeing to pay the agreed-upon fee and acknowledging that they are aware of policies pertaining to fees.

BEFORE MEETING THE CLIENT
Come Prepared

When clients come to see clinicians to discuss highly personal difficulties, they are often anxious. It is our job to keep the tone of our sessions as calm as possible. This can be challenging since there is a lot to remember when you first meet with a client. You need general information on the client (likely collected during an initial phone call), any forms that the client needs to fill out (e.g., consent forms), your assessment measures, pens and pencils, and a watch or clock to help you be mindful of the time. In some settings, you might also need to be prepared to videotape or audiotape your session. Remembering all of these items and tasks can be even harder if you are seeing clients in an office shared by many clinicians, where you do not have all of these items at hand. Running in and out of the office/therapy room to retrieve important papers, tools, or items will likely make you appear disorganized and unprofessional to your client.

A key to being prepared is to give yourself enough time. If you have your first client at 9 A.M. and know that you have to get set up in an office shared by other clinicians, get there a half hour early. Take some time to make sure you have everything that you need and that the office is neat and clean. If you see clients in your own office, organize all the materials that you need and again, be sure that your work area is clean and cleared of any client-related information (e.g., phone messages, files). Clients will rightfully doubt your commitment to confidentiality if they come into your office and easily see the names of other clients on papers scattered around your desk.

Be Mindful of the Focus of Attention

Before moving on to the nuts and bolts of this first in-person interaction, it is worth mentioning the issue of focus of attention. In all of our interactions with clients—assessments or therapy sessions—our attention should be focused on the client. When people are anxious, their tendency is to focus on themselves: "Am I saying the right thing?" "Can the client tell that I've never done this before?" "Did I forget a question in that last section of the assessment?" To some extent, it is important to pay attention to such things in order to make sure that the goals of the session are accomplished. However, too much focus on how you are coming across to the client can be detrimental. It might make you miss out on what the client is saying, or it might actually make it more likely that you will forget to ask something important.

When interacting with clients, we should be focusing as much as possible on them. We should be attending to what they say and to what they are communicating through their body language and facial expressions. This level of attention will allow you to leave the session with the information that you need to make a diagnosis and begin the process of conceptualizing the case.

With this being said, there are appropriate times for being more self-focused. During supervision, you can certainly discuss how you believe you came across during your interactions with a client. It can also be very useful for beginning clinicians to watch (or listen to) their own therapy tapes and identify behaviors that they might want to change. For example, you might see yourself as task-oriented to the exclusion of being empathic toward the client. This knowledge can be useful in future therapy interactions.

IN THE WAITING ROOM

The first place that we typically meet clients face to face is the waiting room. When greeting clients, it is important to put them at ease, while also being mindful of confidentiality. If a receptionist checks clients in, it is best to ask him or her to indicate which client is yours. Then, approach this person, introduce yourself, welcome the client to the clinic, and escort the client to your office. If you must call out a name in the waiting room, sticking to a first name helps to maintain the client's confidentiality.

IN THE ROOM WITH THE CLIENT

In the first few minutes of the initial session, what should be foremost in your mind are social graces. This seems like silly advice—after all, there is a lot of work to get done. Yet we are so often rushing to get tasks accomplished that we forget to greet clients, welcome them to the clinic, ask how they are, and introduce ourselves. These first few moments can make a big difference in establishing rapport, setting clients at ease, and letting them know that we are interested in them as people and not just as clusters of symptoms.

Introductions and Permission to Record

At this point in the session, it is appropriate to ask clients how they are, and it is certainly important to address them correctly (e.g., "Would you like me to call you Mrs. Jones or Susan?"). In general, it is best when you first meet adult clients to call them Mr. or Mrs. X. Many clients will immediately ask that you call them by their first name and it is certainly fine to ask clients if they feel comfortable being addressed in that way. The overarching rule is to have respect for your clients. Although it is our experience that most therapy clients are perfectly fine with being called by their first names, being asked first if this is acceptable shows that we respect their wishes and helps to establish good rapport.

When introducing yourself to clients, provide your name and let them know what they can call you (e.g., whether you like to be addressed as Dr. Smith, Miss Smith, Jane, etc.) You might also want to tell the client a bit about your "professional self." For example, "I've been working at this clinic for about two years. My main interest in both my clinical work and my research is in marital relationships. I've been working with couples since graduate school and really enjoy it a lot." While this discussion of one's professional self is by no means mandatory, it can break the ice and make clients feel more comfortable. Sometimes clients may ask you for more information about yourself. They may be curious and want to know if you are married, have children, where you grew up, as well as other more personal information. Such questions may derive from clients' normal curiosity about their clinicians. They may also ask because it seems to them that the therapeutic relationship is one-sided. They tell us about themselves in great detail while we share relatively nothing about ourselves. Regardless of why clients may ask for more personal details, you may find yourself feeling uncomfortable when pressed for more information. When deciding how to answer such questions, keep in mind that you need to balance the goal of developing therapeutic rapport with the sense of how much is too much self-disclosure. How much is too much may be determined by many things, including your own personal comfort level regarding self-disclosure and, as discussed in greater detail in Chapter 7, whether or not additional self-disclosure to a client is contraindicated. In many cases, though, it may be acceptable to provide some personal detail in order to satisfy a client's curiosity and for the sake of building a strong therapeutic relationship.

One piece of information that you must disclose is your status as a trainee. The APA *Ethical Principles of Psychologists and Code of Conduct* (2002) requires that all clinicians in training tell clients that they have a supervisor and provide them with the supervisor's name (code 10.01c). The Canadian Psychological Association's (CPA) *Code of Ethics for Psychologists* (2000) makes similar requirements (code III.22). In Chapter 7, we discuss additional issues that might relate to telling your clients about your level of training. For the time being, keep in mind that the issue of supervision must be raised early in your initial session with a client.

One final piece of business that must be taken care of before proceeding with the initial session is the issue of audiotaping or videotaping sessions. In research settings, assessments and therapy sessions are typically taped; in clinically oriented settings, trainees are often asked to tape their assessments and therapy sessions for supervision purposes. In gaining permission, clinicians should explain to clients why sessions will be taped, who will have access to tapes, and what precautions will be taken to ensure confidentiality (e.g., how tapes are stored, etc.). In general, most clients express little resistance to being taped after they have been properly briefed on confidentiality and are told how the tapes will be used in supervision.

Giving an Overview of the Session

Once introductions are done, clients should be given an overview of what the session will entail. Generally, in the first meeting, the clinician "takes care of business"—specifically, obtaining consent to do the assessment and discussing confidentiality with the client—and then proceeds to the assessment. In the remainder of this chapter, we discuss how to "take care of business"; in the next chapter, the process of assessment is outlined, including how to initially orient clients to the assessment process.

Taking Care of Business

At the start of the initial session, consent should be obtained and confidentiality discussed. The client should be given ample opportunity to read the consent form (see the next section) and should be invited to ask questions. Respecting clients' concerns and questions during this process can get the therapeutic alliance off to a good start even before clients begin to discuss the difficulties that they are having.

Obtaining Consent for Assessment

For which activities do we need to obtain consent from clients? Both the APA (2002) *Ethical Principles* and the CPA (2000) *Code of Ethics* require psychologists to obtain informed consent for both assessment and therapy (see codes 3.10, 9.03, and 10.01 in the APA code and code I.19 in the CPA code). Furthermore, it is important to obtain consent "as early as is feasible" (APA code 10.01a). In general, written consent is superior to simply recording in a chart that verbal consent was obtained, although the APA and the CPA permit both methods.

There are some key points to keep in mind when obtaining consent. In the case of written consent, it is always a good policy to read through the consent form with the client. However, you certainly can highlight the key points more informally. In either case, clients should always be given the opportunity to read through the consent form at their own pace. Once clients have finished reading, it is important to ask them if they have understood what they have read and to invite them to ask questions. If you sense that clients have not understood the form, it is best to review it with them and put it into language they can understand. If a client immediately jumps to the signature line and starts to sign his or her name without reading the consent form, it is advisable to emphasize the importance of reviewing the form before signing. If consent is being obtained verbally, the key points that would be included in a written consent form should be reviewed with the client and his or her verbal consent should be noted in the chart.

Consent forms should include some essential information, and these essentials are outlined in both the APA and the CPA codes (see code I.24 in the CPA code and 9.03a, 10.01a in the APA code). In general:

1. Clients must understand the *purpose and nature of the activity*. This section of the consent form should outline for clients what the assessment or treatment program will entail and the purpose of these activities. These descriptions should be written and also verbally explained to clients in lay terms.

2. Clients must be informed about likely *benefits and risks* of the activity. Although our natural inclination is to tout all the likely benefits of our activities as clinicians, clients cannot be expected to make informed decisions about assessment and treatment without being aware of both the benefits and the risks. It is definitely appropriate to point out to clients that CBT has garnered a great deal of empirical support and to give them specific information on the problem for which they are seeking help (e.g., in treatment outcome studies, about 75% of clients with social phobia benefit from CBT). On the other hand, clients should be informed that positive outcomes cannot be guaranteed for any one client. It is also appropriate to point out to clients that making the cognitive and behavioral changes that are essential in all CBT programs might, in the short-term, be difficult and stressful.

3. Clients must be told of *alternatives to the activity* (e.g., other treatments) and *likely consequences of nonaction*. Although many clinicians feel committed to the school of treatment to which they subscribe, we are ethically obligated to let our clients know of other treatments that might help them. For example, "If you do not seek treatment for your social anxiety, you might continue to experience difficulties in social situations. Alternative treatments for social phobia are available. Research has shown that certain medications are as effective as CBT in the short-term for the treatment of social anxiety. However, CBT tends to be more effective than medication in the long-term. No other psychological treatments have been shown to be more effective than CBT for the treatment of social phobia."

4. Consent forms must also make clear that clients can *refuse to participate* in the given activity or *withdraw at any time* without prejudice.

5. Consent forms must also include a discussion of *confidentiality protections and limitations*. The issue of confidentiality must be discussed with each and every client prior to the initiation of assessment or therapy.

Discussing Confidentiality

The importance of discussing confidentiality cannot be emphasized enough. Some clients will be very clear with you that this is a concern for them. They might worry about information being released to their family members or to their employers. Even clients who do not come right out and mention concerns about confidentiality might be concerned about it, and rightfully so, given that therapy involves discussing deeply personal matters with a complete stranger. The bottom line is that without the protection of confidentiality, many clients would not consider therapy in the first place or, alternatively, would enter therapy but withhold discussion of issues that might be very relevant to the difficulties they are having.

How can clients be reassured about this very important issue? First, you can tell your clients how important confidentiality is to you and the other staff at your clinic and that you are bound to maintain confidentiality (under most circumstances) not only by ethical codes but also by law. Tell your clients that you will not speak about them with anyone except your supervisor, other clinicians who attend group supervision meetings with your supervisor, or other people at the clinic who are directly involved in their care (e.g., the psychiatrist at your clinic who takes care of medication for clients).

Just as important, you must discuss the specific circumstances under which confidentiality must be broken. These circumstances are mandated by the laws of each state or province and should be clearly understood by both you and each client with whom you work. If you are not aware of the rules, ask your clinical supervisor to explain them or call your state or provincial licensing board and have the information sent to you (see *www.asppb.org* for contact information for all state and provincial licensing boards).

In general, clients should be told that confidentiality will be breached if (1) they threaten to harm themselves; (2) they threaten to harm others; (3) they tell you about the abuse of a child; or (4) their records are subpoenaed by a court of law. Some states and provinces also have other mandatory reporting laws (e.g., mandatory reporting of abuse of adults who cannot protect themselves, etc.). It is worth reemphasizing that a discussion of confidentiality, and limits to it, should occur as early in your contact with the client as possible.

An important issue related to confidentiality arises when you are working for a third party—for example, when you are doing employee assessments for an employer, student assessments for a school district, or assessments that are ordered by the court. In such situations, the rules of confidentiality change. Here, you do not work for the person you are assessing but rather for the employer, the school district, or the court and, as such, they have access to the information that you collect from the client. In these situations, all parties must be made aware of the limits of confidentiality.

Some tips to remember about the process of obtaining consent from clients are summarized in Table 2.1.

THE CASE CONCEPTUALIZATION (THUS FAR)

At this point in your interactions with the client, you have only "taken care of business." You have introduced yourself and discussed your background and training (including informing the client of your trainee status). You have obtained consent for the forthcoming activities and you have carefully outlined confidentiality and limits to it. You, or someone on your clinic staff, has set a fee and discussed with the client rules around collection of fees, missed appointments, and the like. Although you have not yet started to talk with the client about his or her presenting problem, this initial contact will certainly yield important information that may prove useful in your conceptualization of the case as well as in treatment design and implementation.

Beginning clinicians may easily overlook the beginning of the first session, thinking that the real work has yet to begin. However, discussion of these administrative topics can reveal a fair bit. For example, a client might become argumentative during a discussion about fees or the rules of therapy. Another client might be nervous and unassertive during a similar discussion. Clients may also have notable reactions to the discussion of confidentiality. Unusually strong reactions during these informational discussions might lead the clinician to hypothesize that a particular issue is sensitive and should be explored more thoroughly during the assessment process. Client reactions during this time may also provide information about how he or she reacts to interpersonal conflict or difficult issues more generally. The bottom line here is that the observed reactions of clients during initial discussions can be informative for the clinician as they might suggest what to expect in future sessions and in situations outside of therapy when similar and other difficult topics are discussed.

TABLE 2.1. Obtaining Consent

As early as is feasible in your clinical activities with patients, it is essential to obtain consent.

Important points to remember

- Consent must be obtained for assessment and therapy.
- Written consent is superior to oral consent.
- Let clients read through consent forms at their own pace, check that they have understood what they read, and invite questions.

Essential information to cover when obtaining consent

- Clients must understand the *purpose and nature of the activity.*
- Clients must be informed about likely *benefits and risks* of the activity.
- Clients must be told of *alternatives to the activity* (e.g., other treatments) and *likely consequences of nonaction.*
- Consent forms must also make clear that clients can *refuse to participate* in the given activity or *withdraw at any time* without prejudice.
- Consent forms must also include a discussion of *confidentiality protections and limitations.*

Discussing confidentiality

- Reassure clients about how important confidentiality is to you and your clinic staff. Explain to clients that you are bound to maintain confidentiality according to both ethical codes and the law.
- Discuss the specific circumstances under which confidentiality must be broken.
- Discuss the issue of releasing information to third-party payers.

A CASE EXAMPLE

At this point, we introduce a case example as a means of demonstrating the initial contact and the start of the assessment process. After seeing an article in the local newspaper about a treatment clinic, Michael J., a 40-year-old single man, telephoned to inquire about help for social anxiety. The clinic secretary put him through to a clinician after hearing his request for help. During this first phone call, Mr. J. spoke to a clinician at the clinic for approximately half an hour. The clinician first asked him to briefly describe what kinds of difficulties he was having.

Initial Contact

CLINICIAN: What's led you to call our clinic today, Mr. J.?

MICHAEL: Well, I know it sounds dumb for a grown man, but I've been having a lot of problems with speaking up in public. I just went back to school and can't speak up in class, and the work I am doing now requires a lot of public speaking that also makes me feel uncomfortable. I'm always screwing up—it's just terrible.

CLINICIAN: When you're in these situations, what do you fear will happen? What makes you reluctant to speak up in groups?

MICHAEL: It's just this bad feeling. I just feel so nervous.

CLINICIAN: That's what we hear from a lot of our socially anxious clients. Do you have a sense of why it's so bad to feel nervous?

MICHAEL: Well, if I feel nervous, I'm going to look nervous, aren't I? I have to tell you—I blush like no one else on earth. Whenever I speak in public, I feel my face just glowing, burning red. I also know that my voice sounds shaky when I get nervous. It's just terrible.

CLINICIAN: So, it sounds like you're worried about people noticing your physical symptoms of anxiety. Is that right?

MICHAEL: Yeah. I guess.

CLINICIAN: Okay, so if people do notice you blushing or your voice shaking, what might happen?

MICHAEL: Well, they'll just think I'm an idiot. They'll wonder why I ever got into school and whether I will ever be able to manage being a priest.

CLINICIAN: You're becoming a priest?

MICHAEL: Yeah. Pretty interesting job for someone with social anxiety, isn't it?

CLINICIAN: Well, yes . . . and that actually leads to my next question. What sorts of changes would you like to make in your life right now?

MICHAEL: I want to feel more at ease in social situations. I want to be able to pay attention to my work, and not so much to how I am coming across and what people must be thinking of me. It's exhausting.

CLINICIAN: Kind of like your attention is divided?

MICHAEL: Yeah, I am half-focused on work, but half of my mind is always busy thinking about how I am doing. I want to feel 100% focused. I know that isn't completely realistic for someone like me, but I need to be doing better than I am right now. This social anxiety could really jeopardize my career . . . and given the kind of career I am choosing, it could also jeopardize my life.

Making a Recommendation

At the end of this phone call, the clinician concluded that Michael would be a good candidate for a more thorough assessment at the clinic. From their brief discussion, it appeared that Michael met diagnostic criteria for social phobia. He feared that in social and performance situations, he would exhibit signs of anxiety (like blushing and shaking) that would lead people to evaluate him negatively. In order to confirm this diagnosis, a thorough in-person assessment would be necessary and would also allow the clinician to ascertain whether other comorbid conditions were present that might be relevant to the treatment. Michael was also very motivated to engage in treatment at the time that he called the clinic, primarily because his social anxiety was interfering with his career and lifestyle choices. An in-person evaluation would allow the clinician to provide Michael with more information about treatment and how it might be helpful to him. In the case of clients who seem less motivated when they call, an in-person meeting allows the clinician to more thoroughly evaluate whether the time is right for the client to begin treatment. Sometimes clients become more motivated when they hear about the nature of treatment or about successes experienced by other clients.

Michael's initial phone call came to a close with the clinician "normalizing" his concerns, affording him the opportunity to ask questions, and setting up the evaluation.

CLINICIAN: You sound as if you are having concerns very similar to those of clients we treat here. It's impossible to make a diagnosis based on a brief phone call, so if you were interested, the next step would be for you to come in to our clinic to do a more thorough assessment. There are two main components to our assessment process. We send clients some questionnaires that inquire about social anxiety and related issues. We also bring clients into our clinic to meet with one of our clinicians for a clinical interview. At this time, you'll have the opportunity to go into more detail about the difficulties you're having with social anxiety, and the clinician will also inquire about other problems you might be having right now.

MICHAEL: What would happen after all of that? Should I have treatment for this problem?

CLINICIAN: That's an excellent question. The purpose of assessments like the ones we do here are really twofold—to figure out the kinds of difficulties you're having, but also to see whether treatment is necessary, and if so, what that treatment should be. From what you're telling me, it sounds like treatment could be really helpful, but let's hold off on that decision till your assessment is complete. Once we finish the assessment, we'll set a time for you to come back in so that I can give you some feedback and we can discuss recommendations for treatment.

In-Advance Arrangements

At this point, Michael and the clinician set up a 2-hour appointment. This would afford enough time for the clinician to assess the client more thoroughly using the Structured Clinical Interview for the DSM-IV (SCID)—the standard assessment done at the clinic where Michael was seen. The clinician gave Michael directions to the clinic and got his permission and mailing address to send him some questionnaires to complete before coming in for his assessment. He was also asked to speak to the clinic business administrator to discuss fees for the assessment.

The First Visit: Assessment

Michael arrived for his assessment interview a few minutes early. He came with his questionnaires fully completed and cordially greeted the clinician in the waiting room. Michael was dressed nicely and was well groomed. The clinician led him to an interview room. Prior to the appointment, she had set out a copy of the SCID, a pen, and her watch. She also brought in a "cheat sheet" on score interpretations for the measures that Michael had completed at home, as well as a copy of the DSM.

Introductions and Taking Care of Business

Introductions were exchanged and the client asked that he be called Michael. The clinician discussed confidentiality and reviewed the assessment consent form verbally with Michael, answered his questions, and then gave him time to read the consent form to himself. As he read, the clinician reviewed Michael's self-report measures to get an idea of things that might be problematic for him. The only notable findings were relatively high scores on the measures of social anxiety and slightly low scores on a measure of quality of life (indicating slight dissatisfaction). He scored within the nonclinical range on a measure of depression and on measures assessing for the presence of other anxiety-related symptoms, including worry and panic.

Giving an Overview of the Session

Once Michael had signed the consent form, his clinician then proceeded to explain the purpose of the assessment interview and how the rest of the session would proceed, being mindful to help Michael feel comfortable with the whole process.

CLINICIAN: For the rest of today's session, we are going to be doing a structured clinical interview. This interview assesses for a range of different psychological difficulties. It is a way to make sure that we "cover all of our bases." We want to see whether social anxiety is the best explanation for your problems and also whether you are having any other difficulties that we should be aware of. Some of the questions I ask will be very relevant to you, and we will focus on these sections. Other questions won't apply to you, and we'll just move past those sections. The goal of our time together today is to get a sense of the kinds of difficulties that you are having and how we might best go about treating them. How does that sound?

MICHAEL: A little scary. It's kind of hard for me to talk about all of this stuff.

CLINICIAN: I understand completely. Is there anything specifically that is making you feel anxious?

MICHAEL: Well, I think I said to you on the phone that I feel dumb for having social anxiety. I mean, I'm 40 years old. Don't people grow out of this?

CLINICIAN: That's an excellent question. What we know from research on social anxiety is that it tends to start about 20 years before people seek treatment. Many of the socially anxious clients that we see here are right around your age. Simply having social anxiety can make it more difficult to seek treatment than having another anxiety disorder that is not related to fear of being negatively evaluated by others.

MICHAEL: Yeah. I guess I just think you're going to think I'm a freak for having this problem.

CLINICIAN: My job here is to help you, not to judge you. The best way to help me figure out what's causing problems for you and how to help you is to be open and honest and not worry too much about how you are coming across. Why don't we get started with the interview and see how it feels?

At this point, Michael's clinician encouraged him to request a break if he needed one and then progressed into the demographic section of the assessment interview. Let's pause here in the case of Michael. We will return to Michael's interview in Chapter 3 after first discussing assessment goals and methods.

Chapter 3

■ ■ ■

THE PROCESS OF ASSESSMENT

At this point, clients have given consent to participate in the assessment and have been informed about confidentiality and limits to it. Now it is time to move ahead with the assessment. In this chapter, we first offer some general guidelines and then discuss the goals of the assessment process. Next, we discuss how to use various assessment tools to accomplish these goals. Finally, we continue to use the case of Michael J. to give readers a sense of how a typical assessment might proceed.

BEING MINDFUL OF YOUR REACTIONS

During assessments, clients reveal all sorts of information, some of which will be very unusual or upsetting. Clinicians' reactions to information that clients share can significantly affect the therapeutic relationship. If clinicians' reactions reinforce clients' negative beliefs about sharing information with others (e.g., they will think I am odd, they won't want to help me, etc.), clients may (rightfully) feel hesitant to share any more information with the clinician. It is essential to react with sensitivity to what our clients tell us.

Let's discuss the ways in which one should *not* react. It almost goes without saying (although we will say it anyway) that clinicians should not tell clients that their experiences are odd, unusual, or distasteful. What might be more difficult for clinicians is to refrain from subtle reactions that could make clients feel bad. These more subtle reactions might include negative facial expressions or taking a longer than usual time to react to what a client has said or not reacting at all, leaving an uncomfortable silence in the room. Even when clients reveal difficult information, make sure to acknowledge that you have heard them by nodding or by saying, "I see" or "I understand." When clients tell us something very difficult, it can also be beneficial to let clients know that you are glad that they shared this information since it helps you to better understand the experiences that they are having and how to help them.

What clients define as odd or unusual or troubling about themselves will often be "all in a day's work" for clinicians. Although beginning clinicians have not seen many cases, they do possess knowledge from reading, watching tapes of clients, and participating in group supervision meetings where they are exposed to many other cases beyond the ones that they have treated themselves. As we gain more experience, things that clients tell us will map onto things that we have heard from other clients with whom we have worked. Thus, when clients reveal experiences or feelings, we are rarely as shocked as they expect us to be. Clients often feel comforted to know that others experience similar symptoms and that their symptoms can be ameliorated with treatment. With this in mind, a general rule of thumb is to try to normalize clients' difficulties without minimizing them. A phrase like "We see a lot of clients here with concerns like that" can go a long way.

At times, however, we do come across clients whose symptoms or experiences are unique. This leaves us unable to say "Yes, of course I've seen clients with concerns similar to yours." It is often the case, however, that we can draw parallels to similar cases. Consider a client with obsessive–compulsive disorder (OCD) and bulimia nervosa. The client's main OCD symptom was hoarding. While she hoarded items like newspapers and paper cups and rubber bands like many clients do, she also hoarded food. In fact, her entire apartment was filled with bits of food she had picked up here and there. When she engaged in binge eating, this client would binge in part on fresh, newly purchased food, but would also binge on food that she had hoarded that was often rotten and half-eaten by mice. This case was very shocking to the clinician who assessed this client, and at the end of the assessment, the client asked the clinician if she had ever before seen a case like this. In truth, the clinician had not. She said to the client, "I haven't seen a case exactly like yours. But, like all clients with OCD who engage in hoarding, you hold on to stuff because you worry that you might need it in the future. In your case, you hold on to food because you are nervous that you will not have enough food to binge on. This is very similar to clients who hold on to years worth of newspapers because they worry that they might eventually need some of the information that is in them." By responding in this way, the clinician acknowledged that the client's case was unique, but was able to draw parallels with other cases, helping the client to see that she understood her experiences and could devise an effective treatment plan to help her.

One final issue deserves mention. Beginning clinicians often worry about crying in front of clients when they share very painful or frightening stories. One thing to keep in mind is that having an extreme reaction (e.g., tears steaming down your face) is quite unlikely. Our reactions to clients whom we are meeting for the first time will likely be quite different from our reactions to family members or close friends whom we have known for years. Even on this different level, though, therapy is an interpersonal relationship, and having tears well up in reaction to a particularly sad or frightening story is only natural. Clinicians should not be terribly concerned about such a reaction—if anything, it communicates empathy to clients and validates the emotional experience that they had to the event that they are describing. With that being said, clinicians should let their supervisors know if they are regularly having a difficult time remaining composed in therapy sessions. After all, the emotional reaction of the clinician should not draw attention away from the client. Supervisors may be able to offer beginning clinicians some advice on how to best address this kind of difficulty.

THE GOALS OF ASSESSMENT

With the emotional tone for the evaluation set, we now turn to the concrete goals of the assessment process. As we have already noted, two goals should be met over the course of an assessment: (1) arriving at a diagnosis to describe the client's symptoms and (2) arriving at a tentative explanation of the client's symptoms in CBT terms that can then be used to plan treatment. Clients often arrive in our offices with vague problems— they feel down, worried, or stressed out, or are engaging in behaviors that they or others view as problematic. In these situations, it is our job to develop an understanding of the history of the problem and current factors that may explain why the problem persists. Understanding what maintains clients' difficulties allows us to devise a treatment plan aimed at altering these maintaining factors.

TOOLS FOR ACCOMPLISHING ASSESSMENT GOALS

In this section, we will describe tools that can be used for accomplishing the assessment goals. Since the key to doing a complete assessment is gathering information from multiple sources, we will cover a number of assessment tools, including interviews, questionnaires, and behavioral assessments. We also discuss how to go about gathering information from individuals who are familiar with the client's difficulties.

Semistructured Clinical Interviews

The way clinicians go about assessing clients really depends on the setting in which they work, the orientation to which they ascribe, and their own personal style. Regardless of these factors, one of the most popular assessment techniques is the clinical interview. Many clinicians routinely do a clinical interview of some sort in order to identify the difficulties that clients are having and to plan a course of treatment for them.

Interviews vary in the degree to which they are structured. In some settings, particularly those in which research is carried out, semistructured interviews are typically used. Commonly used interviews of this type include the Structured Clinical Interview for DSM-IV (SCID-IV; First, Spitzer, Gibbon, & Williams, 1997) and the Anxiety Disorders Interview Schedule for DSM-IV (ADIS-IV; Brown, DiNardo, & Barlow, 1994). The goal of this kind of interview is to arrive at a diagnosis (or diagnoses) based on current DSM diagnostic criteria.

When novice clinicians first begin using semistructured clinical interviews, they typically have several concerns. Some beginning clinicians may worry that the interview will sound very stilted and impersonal. This is certainly possible, particularly when clinicians are not yet entirely comfortable with the interviews. Beginning clinicians tend to be more wedded to reading questions verbatim (as all clinicians should, in fact, according to the instructions for administering these interviews!) and are often so focused on keeping on track with the interview that they indeed may come across as stilted and not particularly interested in the client.

Rest assured that your interview style will improve over time. As you become more comfortable with these interviews, you will be less focused on keeping track of which questions to ask and more focused on what the client is saying. Once you become comfortable with them, semistructured interviews are not quite as structured as they might seem at first glance. Although questions should be read verbatim, simply reading the written questions to clients will not yield much useful information. It is important to ask follow-up questions that will help you arrive at a decision about whether or not a client indeed meets criteria for a particular disorder.

When using semistructured interviews, it is also essential to be mindful of rapport. As already noted, the tone might be stilted and formal when you are a novice interviewer. After a couple of years of doing clinical interviews, when you can practically recite them in your sleep, you might begin to sound bored and uninterested. To avoid either situation, focus on what the client is *saying*. Although you might be asking the same questions you always ask, you will never get exactly the same reply. Be attentive to what clients are saying, follow-up with questions that are relevant to them, and above all, be warm and empathic. These qualities can turn a potentially staid interview into a very positive experience for clients, during which they feel understood and come to believe that you will be able to offer them some solutions to their distress.

Unstructured Clinical Interviews

In some settings, less importance is placed on whether or not clients meet strict diagnostic criteria for a particular disorder. In fact, many practitioners of various theoretical orientations do not believe in the value of DSM diagnoses (see Sadler, 2002, for a discussion of these issues). Of greater interest to them might be how their clients are functioning across a number of different areas (e.g., family life, work life, etc.) and how clients deal with the challenges of life (e.g., coping style, social support, etc.). In this light, interviews can be less directive and more flexible, while still allowing the clinician to gather sufficient information to understand clients' difficulties and devise a treatment plan.

Unstructured interviews are associated with some unique worries for beginning clinicians. Semistructured interviews, while certainly requiring clinical skill and intuition, provide interviewers with a framework for completing the assessment process. In the unstructured interview, that "crutch" is not there. Or is it? Most clinicians who use unstructured interviews as their primary means of assessment use a standard outline of topics that their interview will follow. In Table 3.1, we have provided a set of guidelines that you might want to follow and then adjust as you develop your own style.

Demographic Information: A Good Starting Point

A good place to start is to gather demographic information. Questions of this nature are usually nonthreatening and help to establish rapport. They can also paint for you a very preliminary picture of how the client is functioning. Of greatest import is the degree to which the client's current difficulties have affected his or her work, educational, or social functioning. You should assess whether the difficulties have recently resulted in a significant change from previous functioning. For example, a mother with small children and a part-time job may tell you that she used to be able to easily balance her family and work responsibilities but that since she started feeling depressed, she finds even the most menial tasks overwhelming. Some clients have never functioned much differ-

TABLE 3.1. Summary of Topics for an Unstructured Clinical Interview

Demographics

- Name; date of birth/age
- Ethnic/religious background
- Current work status/educational status
- Current relationship status/family structure
- Current living arrangements

Presenting problem

- Description of problem
- Onset and course of problem; frequency of symptoms/episodes
- Antecedents of the problem (e.g., situational triggers, life events, etc.)
- Thoughts associated with the problem (e.g., automatic thoughts, beliefs)
- Reactions to the triggers/life events (e.g., emotional, physiological, and behavioral reactions).
- Intensity and duration of the problem
- Previous treatment for the problem
- Additional problems

Family background

- Ages of parents and siblings
- Upbringing and family relations
- Parents' marital history
- Parents' occupations, socioeconomic status
- Family medical and psychiatric history

Personal history

- Developmental milestones
- Early medical history
- Adjustment to school and academic achievement
- Presence of acting out
- Peer relations
- Hobbies/interests
- Dating history

ently than they are currently functioning. In such cases, it is important to assess whether clients are functioning in a way that is congruent with where one would expect them to be in life. For example, it would be notable if a 30-year-old man was still living at home with his parents and had never finished school or held a job.

The Presenting Problem

With this demographic information covered, it is appropriate to ask the client about his or her presenting problem. A good way to ask this question is "What brings you here today?" or "Can you tell me about the problem that you've been having?" Let clients explain their problems in their own words, and as you continue to discuss these issues during the interview, try to use their words. If a client refers to a panic attack as a "stress attack," you may want to ask later in the interview for him to tell you more about his "stress attacks" rather than for him to tell you more about his "panic attacks." In discussing the presenting problem, it is important to get a sense of its history—when it began and what kind of course it has taken. For disorders of an episodic nature (e.g., depression), you should assess how many separate episodes the client has experienced. You can also gather information on the frequency of symptoms (e.g., the number of panic attacks a person has each week, or the amount of time taken up each day by obsessions and compulsions for a client with OCD).

In keeping with the cognitive-behavioral model, there are a number of things that clinicians should learn about a client's presenting problem beyond its onset and course. Looking back at Figure 1.1, clinicians want to start "filling in the blanks" of the cognitive model in order to understand the case. A good place to start is with situations and events that bring on the problematic thoughts and behaviors. Clients can be asked what was going on in their lives immediately before, and in the several months before, a problem began or intensified (e.g., "What was going on in your life before you started feeling depressed?"); which stimuli trigger their current symptoms (e.g., "In what sorts of situations do you experience panic attacks?"); and the larger contexts in which difficulties are experienced.

Clients should then be asked what they think about in these situations. This begins to tap into automatic thoughts and deeper, more long-standing core beliefs. For example, a woman whose depression began following her divorce might report, "I won't ever be happy again." Similarly, a person who experiences panic attacks on subways and trains might report that when she is on trains, she always thinks, "My heart is beating so fast that I am going to have a heart attack." As we have explained, a single situation or event can mean very different things to different people, and time must be spent at this part of the assessment coming to an understanding of the client's unique interpretation.

Based on this interpretation, clients will react to similar situations in very different ways. Therefore, clients should be asked about their emotional, behavioral, and physiological responses to these trigger situations. For example, the client with panic disorder can be asked how she feels and behaves when she thinks that she is going to have a heart attack on the subway. She would likely report that she feels terribly anxious (emotion), that she sweats, shakes, and feels her heart pounding in her chest (physiological response), and that when she feels this way she gets off at the next possible stop (behavior). Similarly, the client who became depressed following her divorce can be asked how she feels and behaves when she has the thought that she will never be happy again. She might report that she feels very sad and angry (emotion) and that she virtually never goes out anymore (behavior) because she is so sure she will have a bad time.

While it is essential to inquire about all of these responses (emotions, physiological responses, and behaviors), it is particularly important to spend time talking to clients about escape and avoidance behaviors, since these will be the target of most behavioral work in CBT. To tap into this, clients can be asked, "What sorts of things are you *not* doing right now because of your difficulties?" and "What do you do to try to make your situation more manageable?" While some behavioral responses will be quite obvious (e.g., "I don't ride on subways anymore at all," "I never go out with friends anymore since my divorce"), others will be more subtle, and time should be spent gathering this very important information. For example, our client with panic might get off the train several stops early and walk if she is feeling anxious, or might only get on the subway accompanied by someone who could help her if she were to have a heart attack, or might only ride the subway if she has a cell phone with her and some antianxiety medication. This sort of information is essential to conceptualizing the case and making a plan for treatment.

Before moving on to other problems that clients have, it is also important to ask about treatment that they have received in the past for their difficulties and evaluate the adequacy of the treatment (e.g., Did they receive the right kind of therapy or medication for their difficulties? Did they get an adequate dose of medication? Did they stay in therapy for an adequate period of time?) This information can assist treatment planning. For example, if a client had a full and well-delivered course of CBT in the past and found it to be effective, some booster sessions may be an efficient way to deal with a recurrence of symptoms. Information about treatment history may also be helpful in dealing with clients' beliefs about subsequent therapy. For example, a client with a fear of flying may tell you that he is worried that nothing can help him since past treatment has always been a complete failure. Upon probing, you may learn that he spent a few years in psychodynamic therapy that was not targeted at his fear of flying. It would then be useful to share with the client our knowledge about treating flying phobias, letting him know that he has not yet tried the treatments that have evidence in support of their effectiveness.

Additional Problems

It is also very important to ask clients if they have any problems in addition to their most pressing problems. At this point in the interview, it may be helpful to run through some screening questions for psychiatric disorders, similar to those used in semistructured interviews. Using the DSM as a guide, clients should be asked about difficulties with mood disorders, anxiety disorders, eating disorders, and substance use, as well as somatic concerns (e.g., hypochondriasis, body dysmorphic disorder) and sexual/gender identity concerns. Screening should also be done for psychotic symptoms. As noted earlier, clinicians will develop their own style over time and may become accustomed to screening for other types of difficulties that do not fit neatly into DSM diagnostic categories, like anger problems, perfectionism, and body image concerns. When specific problems are identified, CBT clinicians can again use the cognitive model as a guide to adequately gather information for cognitive-behavioral case conceptualization and treatment planning.

Family Background

Once you have a clear sense of the presenting problem and any other difficulties the client is experiencing, it can be useful to gather information on family background and personal history. This may include information on family socioeconomic status, parents' occupations, family psychiatric and medical history, and family relationship dynamics. This information may provide important clues as to the etiology of an identified problem.

Furthermore, inquiring about family history can help the clinician begin to get a sense of a client's core beliefs. As you may recall from Chapter 1, core beliefs are beliefs about oneself, other people, and the world that form during childhood based on the experiences that we have as we are growing up. Briefly inquiring about our clients' lives as they were growing up can shed some light on the beliefs that underlie their current difficulties. If our recently divorced client grew up in a home where she was constantly told that she could not do anything right, she might see her divorce as yet another personal failure and might see her future as hopeless. This interpretation would be very different from that of a person who grew up in a very loving household. If this person were to get divorced, she might be more able to picture meeting someone new, establishing a strong relationship, and eventually being happy again.

The beliefs that clients hold about the difficulties that they are having can also be related to the beliefs held by their families of origin. Clinicians should inquire about beliefs held by the family about the etiology of mental illness and about the potential effectiveness of therapy, since these will influence the client's own expectations about being able to make positive changes in therapy. If a family member had a similar problem and did very well after treatment, clients might feel quite hopeful about pursuing treatment themselves. If clients observed the converse in their family—namely, an individual who was chronically impaired—they might feel less hopeful about their own prospects for change. They might hold a core belief "I am flawed" or "I am abnormal." When clinicians know about these beliefs, they can help clients to clear up misconceptions that can stand in the way of engaging in the therapy process.

Mental Status Exam

If, after conducting an initial interview, you are in doubt about the client's psychiatric status or you are suspicious about the possibility of an organic brain disorder, you may wish to conduct a Mental Status Exam (MSE). According to Kaplan, Sadock, and Grebb (1994), the MSE "is the description of the patient's appearance, speech, actions, and thoughts during the interview" (p. 276). The MSE can be performed efficiently based on observations made over the course of the assessment, yielding a "sum total of the examiner's observations and impressions of the psychiatric patient at the time of the interview" (p. 276).

The mental status exam is described slightly differently by different authors. In Table 3.2, we outline Kaplan et al.'s format and note things to look out for during the assessment in order to gather the necessary information.

Other Tools: Using Multiple Sources of Information to Round Out the Assessment

While the interview is a part of virtually every psychological assessment, other sources of information can greatly enhance the quality of the assessment. Such sources include self-report questionnaires, observational techniques, client self-monitoring, speaking with other professionals, speaking with other people in clients' lives, and finally, learning from clients' in-session behaviors.

Self-Report Questionnaires

Questionnaires should never be relied on as the sole means of making a diagnosis or formulating a case. Yet, they can certainly be a useful component of the overall assessment process. As we have noted earlier, clients can be asked to complete questionnaires prior to the beginning of the assessment session or can be asked to complete them once the assess-

TABLE 3.2. The Mental Status Exam

General description

• Appearance	How is the client dressed and groomed? How is the client's posture?
• Behavior and psychomotor activity	Is the client exhibiting psychomotor retardation or agitation? Does the client have any unusual motor behaviors like tics, mannerisms, rigidity?
• Attitude toward examiner	How did the client behave toward the clinician? How was the level of rapport between clinician and client?

Mood and affect

• Mood	Did the client speak voluntarily about feelings? What was the depth and intensity of the client's feelings? Were there frequent fluctuations in mood during the interview?
• Affect	Was the client emotionally responsive (inferred from facial expression, tone of voice, etc.) during the interview? Was affect congruent with mood?
• Appropriateness	Were the client's emotional responses congruent with the topic being discussed?

Speech	How was the quantity, rate of production, and quality of the client's speech?

Perceptual disturbances	Did the client experience hallucinations or illusions? If so, what sensory system did they involve?

Thought

• Process or form of thought	Did the client exhibit an overabundance or poverty of ideas? Could the client follow the questions that were asked and answer appropriately?
• Content of thought	Did the client experience delusions? Was there anything else remarkable about the content of thoughts such as obsessions, preoccupations, suicidal or homicidal thoughts, etc.?

Sensorium and cognition

• Alertness and level of consciousness	Did the client exhibit reduced awareness of the environment?
• Orientation	Was the client oriented to time, place, and person?
• Memory	How was the client's recent memory (e.g., what did he or she have for breakfast?) How about his or her remote memory (e.g., memories from childhood)? Did the client do anything to try to conceal cognitive impairments (e.g., confabulation)?

- Concentration and attention — Was the client's concentration impaired during the interview? Did it seem to be due to anxiety/mood disturbance or due to a disturbance in consciousness or a learning deficit?

- Capacity to read and write — Could the client read and write a simple sentence?

- Visuospatial ability — Could the client copy a simple figure?

- Abstract thinking — Could the client think in an abstract way?

- Fund of information and intelligence — Can the client accomplish mental tasks that would be expected for a person of his or her educational level and background?

Impulse control — Can the client control sexual, aggressive, and other impulses?

Judgment and insight — Did the client exhibit capacity for social judgment? To what degree was the client aware of his or her illness and how well did he or she understand the illness?

Reliability — How accurately was the client able to report his or her situation?

Note. Adapted from Kaplan, Sadock, and Grebb (1994, p. 276). Copyright 1994 by Lippincott Williams & Wilkins. Adapted by permission.

ment is over. When questionnaires are given in advance of the assessment session, they can be used during the session to facilitate discussion. Clients might feel reluctant to reveal personal information when we first meet them. While it is our job to establish a strong rapport that makes clients feel more comfortable about revealing things to us, questionnaires can help. For example, a client might deny suicidal thoughts during the assessment interview, but might endorse a self-report item about suicidal ideation. The clinician can bring this up in a sensitive manner: "On the questionnaires that you completed, you noted that you were having some thoughts about suicide. A lot of clients that we see here have a hard time talking about these concerns. Can you tell me a bit more about the kinds of thoughts you've been having recently?"

Keep in mind that if you are planning to use questionnaires during the assessment session, it is important that you know how to score them correctly. Furthermore, you must know what the score means and how it can be used in a clinically useful way. If you use a standard battery of measures, you can create a "cheat sheet," noting scoring rules and the meaning of specific ranges of scores.

Even when self-reports are not used to facilitate discussion during the session, they yield extremely useful information that can be integrated into psychological reports. In many cases, self-reports give confirmation of what was learned during the interview. For example, a report might read, "Diagnostic criteria were met for major depressive disorder. The client also reported symptoms of depression on her questionnaires. Her score on the Beck Depression Inventory—II was indicative of moderate depression."

Discrepancies between Interviews and Self-Report Questionnaires

Sometimes clients' questionnaire responses will be incongruent with how they behave. There are many possible explanations for this. Some clients, particularly when they first seek help, might have difficulty articulating exactly what is troubling them. This becomes easier after they have received some psychoeducation and have done some self-monitoring, thereby increasing their own awareness of their problematic thoughts and behaviors.

Other clients might respond to questionnaires in a way that makes them seem far more impaired or far less impaired than they appeared during the interview. For example, a client might appear very emaciated but report very minimal symptoms on a measure of eating and body image disturbance. Similarly, a client might report moderate symptoms of depression during the clinical interview but then score in the severe range on a depression questionnaire. There are various ways to deal with these problems. One is to simply note the inconsistencies in the assessment report. Another is to question clients about these inconsistencies. We certainly do not want to take an accusatory stance, making clients feel as if we are trying to catch them in the act of cheating. It can be useful, however, to ask clients to address these inconsistencies in order to help you to better understand their situation. Clients who underreport or deny symptoms are sometimes not ready for treatment. This is important information and should be taken into account when formulating a plan for the client. Other clients overreport because they are desperate for people to see just how distressed they are or because they seek some other secondary gain (i.e., disability payments). These clients can benefit from some reassurance from the clinician that he or she recognizes their distress and will try to get the help that they need as soon as possible.

Learning from In-Session Behaviors

Careful observation of the client's behavior *during* the assessment is also a valuable source of information for rounding out your case conceptualization. Beyond the client's answers to questions, the way he or she behaves in the room with the clinician can be a window into how he or she behaves and relates to others in "real life." Furthermore, some of these subtleties can help you to see how therapy might progress.

Is the client quiet, reserved, and reluctant to reveal information even as the assessment session progresses? Does he or she become angry as you ask questions? Are there numerous topics that are "off limits"? Does the client flirt with you or ask you questions of a very personal nature? Is the client unhappy with having been assigned a young clinician? Is the client hypercritical of you or of the therapeutic process? There are innumerable ways that a client can behave during an assessment, and these behaviors should be used in conceptualizing the case.

Depending on the client's presenting problem, more formal observation may be used as another assessment option. As the name implies, observation affords the opportunity to see the client's difficulties "in action." How this is accomplished can vary. When people present with relationship difficulties, couples can be observed as they discuss, and try to solve, a problem. If a client presents with a specific phobia, a clinician can set up a behavioral test to see how closely the individual can approach the feared stimulus. For example, if a client fears spiders, the clinician can set up increasingly frightening tasks (e.g., looking at a picture of a spider, touching a picture of a spider, being in a room with a spider that is in a jar, touching the spider, etc.) and see how far the client can progress through these tasks until anxiety prevents him or her from going further. Behavioral tests can also be used to discover whether clients' accounts of their own behavior are biased. For example, in the case of social phobia, clients can be asked to have a casual conversation with a stranger to determine whether they truly do perform poorly in social situations or whether they simply perceive this to be the case. Basically, observation can be used whenever clinicians believe that they will better understand the client if they are able to see his or her difficulties in action. Although behavioral tests can be time consuming and, in some cases, difficult to set up, they can provide much useful information.

Self-Monitoring

Self-monitoring is another excellent way to gain perspective on how clients' difficulties affect their lives on a daily basis. With this technique, the client keeps a record of the occurrence of target behaviors (e.g., nightmares, angry outbursts, etc.). Such recording often includes the date and time of the occurrence, the situation during which the symptom was apparent, thoughts at the time that the symptom occurred, and the client's emotional reactions during the occurrence of the symptom. The information obtained by self-monitoring (e.g., symptom triggers, avoidance, dysfunctional thoughts, and reaction patterns) can be used in the assessment process to more accurately conceptualize the case and to decide how to go about treating it.

Take, for example, a 16-year-old client who presented for treatment of hair pulling (trichotillomania). When this client came in, she had large bald spots on her head, but when asked about how often she pulled her hair or what conditions triggered her hair pulling, she replied that she just was not sure. To obtain better information, the client was sent home to monitor her hair pulling for a week. When she returned for the remainder of her assessment, she showed her clinician her monitoring chart. The client reported that she only pulled during the day at school, and, furthermore, that she only pulled during social studies and driver's education. Her clinician asked her what these two classes had in common, if anything. The client replied that both were terribly boring. During her more interesting and challenging classes, she rarely, if ever, pulled her hair. Her self-monitoring also revealed that hair pulling initially made her feel more awake (e.g., it kept her from falling asleep in boring classes), but that later on she would feel very bad that she had pulled. Finally, her self-monitoring forms also revealed that she was pulling about 150 hairs per week. Knowing where the pulling occurred and the conditions under which it was maintained was crucial for treatment planning. Furthermore, when the client realized how much she was pulling and when she realized that hair pulling was associated with negative affect and thoughts about herself, she felt motivated for treatment despite being forced by her mother to come for the initial assessment.

Speaking to Other Professionals

Before speaking with other professionals about a client's case, the client must give permission. Clinicians should explain in an easily understandable way why they would like to speak to these other professionals and, if clients are amenable, a permission form must be signed and then delivered to the other professional before such conversations can take place. Keep in mind that information should be transmitted in such a way as to maintain confidentiality. Faxes and e-mail messages, while being very convenient modes of communication, can be risky in terms of confidentiality, since both can end up in the wrong hands. Before using either, check with the staff at the clinic in which you work, as well as with local and federal regulations.

Many beginning clinicians feel anxious about contacting other professionals, fearing that they will come across to the other, more experienced professionals as incompetent. Furthermore, beginning clinicians often expect other professionals to be unreceptive. The first thing to keep in mind is that you might be regarded as incompetent if you do *not* consult with other professionals. After all, they possess valuable knowledge that will help you to better treat your clients. Furthermore, most professionals are happy to share their knowledge. Other clinicians often like to talk about their experiences treating clients and ideas that they have for further treatment. Professionals who possess expertise that you do not possess (e.g., physicians, vocational counselors, etc.) are typically receptive to explaining unfamiliar information to you.

On occasion, we come across other professionals who are quite unreceptive; they do not return phone calls or do so in a very gruff and unhelpful manner. For young clinicians, this can be interpreted as a personal affront. Students may assume (and may be right in so assuming) that if their supervisor called this same colleague, the conversation would be much more fruitful. Some people, however, are unhelpful no matter who calls. At such times, it is best to shrug off your interpersonal concerns and focus on getting as much information as you can even if the situation is unpleasant.

With this being said, speaking to other professionals can be very helpful in the assessment process. Sometimes we need to seek input from other health care professionals besides clinicians. This might arise if clients are unclear about the medications that they have taken or are currently taking or if there are questions about the relationship between their physical and mental health. For example, some psychological symptoms (e.g., depression and anxiety) can be explained by medical conditions (e.g., endocrine abnormalities), and it can be helpful to consult with a client's physician with respect to these issues. Some psychological conditions can directly impact a client's physical health (e.g., eating disorders, substance use problems), and it is beneficial to the client in these cases for the clinician to be in touch with the individuals looking after the client's physical health (e.g., primary care physicians, dieticians, etc). Finally, some medical conditions might have an impact on decisions about treatment. For instance, prior to doing interoceptive exposure exercises (exercises that are meant to bring on the symptoms of panic) with a client who has panic disorder and a medical condition like asthma or heart disease, it is wise to check with the client's physician about which exercises are safe to do.

It is also good practice to speak to other professionals who have assessed or treated the individual whom you are assessing. When a client is referred to you, it is often the case that they know why they have been referred (e.g., "I went to be assessed by Dr. X. and he said I needed help with depression, and he said your clinic is the best in the city for that problem"). At other times, clients are less sure about why they have been sent to you, and it can be useful to be in touch with the referring individual to obtain more information.

Sometimes referrals are made when a clinician finishes working on one issue with a client and feels that he or she needs help in another area in which the clinician does not specialize. Perhaps a clinician treated a client successfully for depression, but the client then needs to deal with marital problems. At other times, clinicians of one orientation will refer a client to clinicians of a differing orientation if they believe it to be more suitable to the client and/or the kinds of difficulties that he or she is having. It can be perplexing when you are asked to treat a client by a clinician who has already tried to treat the target problem using the same treatment techniques as you would use. This begs the question of whether your work with the client would make a difference. At times, it might. There are many variables that influence whether a clinician and client work well together, and sometimes one clinician can help a client to progress when another clinician could not. It is always useful in these situations to speak to the other individual who treated the client.

Consider a client who came to be assessed for treatment of OCD. At the time of the assessment, the client was already being seen at another clinic known to do good exposure and response prevention therapy (EX/RP) for OCD. We wondered why this client had not succeeded at EX/RP at the other clinic; when we asked the client, she said that she never did exposure therapy with her other clinician. This seemed curious to us, so we contacted the client's clinician to see how the treatment had progressed. The clinician informed us that the client completely refused to do exposures, despite being provided with a clear rationale for why they were so important to getting past the OCD. When we spoke to the client further about OCD treatment at our clinic, we were clear that treatment would be very similar to that done with her other clinician and asked her if she could imagine doing some of the exposures that we believed would be important for her. We explained that we would do these exposures gradually, only after sufficient education about why they were being recommended. We also asked the client if she would like to speak to some former clients who had felt doubtful about EX/RP at the start of treatment, but who ended up doing very well once they decided to try it. The client said that she would never consider doing such things and did not believe that anyone could convince her to do it. Following this discussion, we referred her to a psychiatrist to discuss medication treatment options and left open the possibility of coming to see us in the future if her willingness to try EX/RP changed. By speaking to this client's former clinician, we were able to address the client's concerns in an up-front and honest way, providing her with information to make a good decision about treatment. Had we not spoken to her former clinician, it was likely that the client would have come to therapy and had another negative experience. Rather, we left the door open for her to come back and start when she was ready, increasing her chance of success.

Speaking to Other People in the Client's Life

Other people in the client's life are another source of useful information. This could include parents, spouses, roommates, and, in the case of younger clients, teachers. The premise behind seeking this sort of information is not to "check up on a client," but rather to help paint a more complete and accurate picture of the client's difficulties.

When other sources are used, it is again crucial to obtain permission. You should never speak to a family member without the client's explicit consent—even telling a family member that the adult client came to be assessed by you is a breach of confidentiality. In gaining permission, clients should be clearly informed as to why you think it would be helpful to speak with these other individuals. For example, consider a client with sleeping problems who has difficulty sleeping at night, but then dozes off during the day. He may have difficulty reporting how often he dozes off and for how long he sleeps when it happens. Consulting with the client's wife and asking her what she has observed will likely yield useful information.

In what context should these conversations occur? If a family member or close friend accompanies the client to the assessment, they can simply be invited to come into the room and contribute to the assessment with the client present. If this is not possible, the discussion can be held on the phone. Regardless of the setting, when speaking to other individuals in clients' lives, it is essential to respect their privacy. These conversations are not an opportunity for you to tell the family member everything the client said during the interview or about your conceptualization of the case ("I think his extreme perfectionism must have to do with what a demanding mother you were when he was growing up"). Remember that these conversations can affect your rapport with the client. If a client goes home from his session and his mother yells at him for saying nasty things about her to his clinician, the client could very well feel angry at the clinician. Rather, you should contact significant others with targeted questions that will help you to conceptualize the case. For example, if a perfectionistic client is having a difficult time describing how his perfectionism affects his life, you might have a discussion with his wife. You could ask her how long he spends cleaning up the house each day and also how he reacts when things around the house are perceived as imperfect.

Ending with a Preliminary Problem List

In the next chapter we introduce Jacqueline Persons's approach to case conceptualization—the process of coming to an initial understanding of a case once the assessment is complete. Persons suggests that a problem list should be created at the end of the assessment as a starting point for the case conceptualization. She describes the problem list as an "all-inclusive list of the client's difficulties" (p. 19). In other words, it serves as a summary of all of the key concerns raised by the client during the assessment process. The problem list includes not only those concerns associated with seeking treatment, like depression, panic attacks, and binge eating, but also such issues as unemployment, marital conflict, and medical problems. Although some of these problems might not appear to be pertinent to therapy, they may very well be. These kinds of problems can precipitate and/or maintain other difficulties; for example, marital problems can precipitate binge eating as a form of emotion regulation; unemployment can play a role in the maintenance of depression. These problems can certainly interfere with treatment (e.g., an unsupportive, critical spouse can impede a client's attempts to regularly engage in exposures to feared situations). After the assessment session is over, the clinician can use this list to begin building a case conceptualization, with the aim of figuring out how these seemingly disparate problems might fit together.

COMMON CONCERNS OF BEGINNING CLINICIANS

Pauses and Breaks

Assessments can be anxiety provoking for beginning clinicians. Many beginning clinicians worry about uncomfortable pauses or silences during the assessment because they might need to take a minute to find their page in an interview, reflect on whether or not they need to probe more about a specific problem, or think about what to ask the client next. Usually the concern is that pausing will cause clients to view the clinician as inexperienced or unable to figure out their problems. Keep in mind that these pauses are likely more noticeable to you than to the client. When pauses are noticed by clients, many will assume that the clinician is thinking—and when clients come to seek help for a problem that is confusing to them, it is unlikely that they will be critical of a clinician who takes a moment or two to mull it over.

Oftentimes, beginning clinicians find themselves perplexed by a particular client. Sometimes this occurs when clients behave in such a way that carrying out the assessment is difficult. They might refuse to talk, or they might speak in a very disorganized manner, or they might deny having any problems at all. At other times, beginning clinicians might be stymied by very complicated cases and might feel that they are simply unable to determine a client's proper diagnosis or which variables may be important for treating a particular client. Small pauses can turn into long gaps in the assessment, and these can certainly become uncomfortable for both client and clinician. In this situation, it is fine in many settings to tell the client that you will take a short break. Offer the client the opportunity to use the washroom, get a snack, or stretch his or her legs. This affords you the opportunity to consult with colleagues, look something up in your DSM, or simply sit and take stock for a few minutes in order to decide how to proceed. Few clients will be bothered by a short break and, in fact, many will be appreciative of it, particularly during long assessments.

Missing a Detail

Another major concern of beginning clinicians is that they will forget to ask a client something important. This realization can strike when preparing your report or preparing to discuss the case in supervision or in a clinic meeting. Colleagues might ask you questions that would aid in conceptualizing the case, and you realize that you simply did not gather the appropriate information to answer them. What can you do? It is not unheard of to phone clients and ask them a few clarifying questions or even call clients in for another meeting. Although beginning clinicians might fear looking incompetent, clients typically interpret this as concern and a desire to better understand the client.

One caveat deserves mention here. Beginning clinicians who are highly anxious might be tempted to frequently phone clients to ask additional questions or call them in to further discuss their case. If you find that you are doing this often, it should be brought up with your supervisor. He or she can help you to figure out why you are "backtracking" so frequently. In some cases, it might be a lack of proficiency. Not knowing the diagnostic criteria or the structure of your assessment instruments might lead you to overlook certain details or forget to ask important questions. This can easily be remedied by additional preparation, observation of more experienced clinicians, and discussion with supervisors and colleagues. Another helpful tip is for clinicians to try to stay focused on what the client is saying during the assessment. Often, beginning clinicians are so focused on seeing if clients meet criteria for particular disorders that they do not ask appropriate questions to really understand clients' histories and what is maintaining their difficulties.

In other cases, clinicians might have unreasonable expectations of what they need to know after an initial assessment. Although it is certainly important to gather sufficient information to conceptualize the case and devise a plan for treatment, be mindful that case conceptualization is an ongoing process. Initially, there might be gaps in your understanding and, in this light, it is completely reasonable that your conceptualization of cases will change as you get to know clients better and as they begin to make changes in their lives.

Making Mistakes

A concern that is related to missing information is the fear of making mistakes. Simply put, beginning clinicians are often fearful of assigning clients the "wrong" diagnosis or conceptualizing their cases incorrectly. For example, a clinician might worry about making errors in differential diagnosis or in deciding which problem to focus on first when a client presents with multiple difficulties. All clinicians will make "incorrect" decisions from time to time. Certainly, this is more often the case with clinicians who are less experienced, but even later in one's career, most clinicians have had the experience of figuring out a few sessions into therapy that they had been off the mark with their assessment of a client.

Beginning clinicians should remember that supervision is in place to catch such errors. Diagnostic decisions and treatment plans are typically discussed before therapy begins. Therefore, any problems can be resolved and therapy can begin on the right course. Although making errors can be embarrassing, it provides important opportunities for learning. Instead of focusing on the short-term discomfort of feeling embarrassed when errors are pointed out to you, focus on the long-term gain in knowledge that will help you the next time you see a similar clinical presentation.

Moving beyond simple diagnoses, beginning clinicians also worry about incorrectly conceptualizing cases. Keep in mind that our initial conceptualization is based on what we learn in our first contact with clients. It is our job to gather enough information to form an understanding of what difficulties clients are having and what is maintaining these difficulties over time. This information helps us to devise a treatment plan, which is always based on a limited amount of data. As we get to know clients better, it is reasonable (and expected) that we will make adjustments to the way that we think about and manage cases.

MICHAEL'S ASSESSMENT INTERVIEW

At the end of Chapter 2, we left our sample client Michael J. just as the clinician was about to begin the assessment interview. We return to him now as the clinician begins with collection of demographic information.

Demographic Information

Michael was a 40-year-old, Caucasian male, raised Catholic in a midsized city in another state. Michael excelled in academics and began medical school at age 20, deciding to become a pathologist. Michael finished his training at age 28, securing a job in the pathology department of an academic medical center. Throughout medical school he had been very involved in the Roman Catholic Church, attending services each Sunday and volunteering at the church soup kitchen and with the youth group. At age 36, he attended a religious retreat during which he felt a calling to become a priest. He spent the last few years exploring this avenue, finally taking a leave of absence from his job 4 months earlier to enter his novitiate year, during which he would consider whether to take his vows as a Catholic priest.

At the time of the assessment, Michael was living in a Catholic seminary where he was taking classes and doing religious work. Prior to coming to the seminary, he lived alone. During his adult years, he dated sporadically and had never had what he considered to be a "serious relationship."

Michael's parents were still living in his hometown. Both were in good health with no history of psychological problems. Despite being faithful Catholics, Michael explained that both were alarmed at his decision to give up a career in medicine and consider the priesthood. He explained that his mother, in particular, was upset at the prospect that he might not marry and have children. His younger sister had been married since she was 21 and was the mother of four.

Presenting Problem and Its History

Michael was asked to briefly describe what led him to contact the clinic. He explained that he had been socially anxious for as long as he could remember. He recalled having always been concerned about blushing. Being very fair-skinned, Michael's ears and face turned quite red when he was feeling anxious. He recounted that during the third grade, he had to give a book report and one of the boys in his class held up a picture of a boy doing a book report with a tomato for a head. Michael said that since that time, he was terrified of public speaking. In high school, he often asked teachers if he could do his presentation one on one instead of in front of the class. Michael said he got away with this most of the time because he was very bright and the teachers actually enjoyed the opportunity to speak in greater depth with him about topics that he was studying. He explained that he did not worry about presenting in front of the teachers since they so clearly valued his intellect over the how he looked.

As a chemistry major in college, Michael was able to get through his undergraduate education without much exposure to public speaking, but social anxiety became an issue for him again in medical school, where students were often put on the spot with questions. Michael also experienced a great deal of anxiety interacting with patients and decided that pathology would be a good field for him, given the limited interaction with other physicians and patients. As in high school, Michael was able to function quite well without social anxiety causing too much trouble for him. Since entering the seminary, however, public speaking became an almost daily task. Students were called on frequently in class, and part of their education was officiating in church services and religious ceremonies. Michael also explained that the frequent interactions with other clergy and parishioners were very difficult for him.

Michael was very open in describing his presenting problem and its history. Furthermore, as he described his difficulties, his clinician asked him questions that would allow her to "fill in the blanks" of the cognitive model. Clearly, the situation that most often brought on Michael's anxiety was public speaking. Throughout his life, more casual social interactions had also been problematic, but to a lesser extent than public speaking. When asked about his thoughts when faced with public speaking, Michael reported: "Everyone notices how red I get" and "When they notice this, they'll *know* I'm incompetent." This led Michael primarily to avoid public speaking (behavioral response), but when he did have to do it (as he had since entering the seminary), he overprepared (behavioral response), became very anxious (emotional response), and experienced many physical symptoms of anxiety, including blushing, shaking, and sweating. As we will demonstrate in the next chapter, during the time Michael's clinician spent with him, she also gathered additional information that helped round out her conceptualization, including getting a sense of the kind of core beliefs that might have been driving his current difficulties.

Semistructured Clinical Interview

The SCID proceeded quite quickly for Michael, who had never experienced many of the symptoms about which he was asked. Michael had a succinct response style—while it was clear that he was listening to each question and considering it, he was able to answer "no" to symptoms he had not experienced without much elaboration. During the section on social anxiety, Michael was very open and able to provide sufficient information for his clinician to make an accurate diagnosis of social phobia (which his clinician already suspected, based on their more open-ended conversation earlier in the meeting). At the end of the interview, it was evident that social phobia was the only current diagnosis for which diagnostic criteria were met. The entire assessment took about 2 hours to complete.

Self-Report Questionnaires

As noted earlier, the clinician had looked over Michael's self-report questionnaires as he read and signed his consent form. These measures were completely congruent with the information provided by Michael during the SCID. Michael reported experiencing moderately severe social anxiety and described some dissatisfaction with his quality of life. At the end of the interview, the clinician queried Michael about the items that he had endorsed on the quality of life measure: dissatisfaction with work and family life. This information would be very beneficial in terms of understanding the case and making recommendations for treatment. One factor for Michael's dissatisfaction with work was obviously social anxiety; his discomfort in many of his new roles made it difficult for him to enjoy the work that he was doing. Another factor was his continuing uncertainty about whether or not to enter the priesthood. He had enjoyed his work in medicine and had taken a year's leave to attend the seminary. Michael expressed concern that a year might not be enough to make this major decision, but knew that he could not spend more than 1 year away from medicine.

Michael also expressed some dissatisfaction with his family and social life. Despite their strong religious faith, Michael's family had been relatively unsupportive of his choice to enter the seminary. Michael explained that he felt that he had lost his right to lean on his family members during this stressful time. In the past, they had always been an amazing source of support, and now he felt "alone, except for God." Michael's clinician asked how he felt about not having a family of his own if he entered the priesthood. Michael replied, "Yeah, I guess that bothers me. It's something I always thought I'd have. But, that is what God asks of us." It was quite clear that Michael was not willing to go into much more detail than that.

Creating the Problem List

As Michael's assessment neared its close, his clinician introduced the concept of the problem list to him:

CLINICIAN: Michael, I'd like to spend a few minutes now summarizing what we have discussed today. In doing this, we are going to create what we call a "Problem List." This list will really help us to take a look at all the difficulties you're facing right now and will help us to understand the "big picture" and map out a plan for treatment.

MICHAEL: That's going to be quite the list.

CLINICIAN: Well, let's start and we'll see. Seems like the first problem we want on there is social anxiety, right?

MICHAEL: Yup. That's the big one.

CLINICIAN: Right. And that's the one we'll likely spend the most time working on. But we also want to consider other issues you are facing, since they may be related to the social anxiety in some meaningful way.

MICHAEL: Right. So, I guess we should put on "career decisions."

CLINICIAN: Exactly. And, how about some of the conflicts you are having with your family right now?

MICHAEL: That's another. Yes, let's put it on there.

CLINICIAN: The one other thing that seems relevant to me is the decision not to have a family of your own if you enter the priesthood.

MICHAEL: You know, I don't think I am going to want to talk about that. This is just something you accept when you are called to serve the Lord.

CLINICIAN: I respect that completely. But it seems to me like an awfully hard decision, even if you do have an incredibly strong sense of faith.

MICHAEL: Of course it's hard.

CLINICIAN: Well, here's what I suggest. Why don't we put it on the problem list, and then see if it comes up as we go along. I won't force any topics on you, and certainly our prime concern is dealing with the social anxiety. But, it seems to me that these other issues might all be related in some way. So, having all the issues down on our list might help us to better make sense of the problems you are currently having.

MICHAEL: That sounds okay with me.

CLINICIAN: Great.

Ending the Session

At this point, the clinician told Michael that they would discuss his case in more detail at the feedback session the following week once she had a chance to more carefully consider his case and review it with her colleagues.

CLINICIAN: Michael, that brings us to the end of our interview today. I'm really glad that you came in to see us. It is pretty clear to me that social anxiety is the major difficulty that you've been having. You've been able to keep it under wraps pretty well these past few years, but this shift in your career and life plans seems to have thrown you for a loop. Is that right?

MICHAEL: Absolutely. Some days it is so tempting to go back to my lab and my apartment and having my family be fine with my choices. You know?

CLINICIAN: I understand completely. Your situation is really interesting because you are going through this major life transition. It seems to me that social anxiety makes these decisions that much harder, doesn't it?

MICHAEL: Yes. It's really confusing. Some days, I think I made a mistake choosing this path. But then I don't know if it's because of the social anxiety or because I really made a mistake. It's so hard. And right now, the only people I can talk to are people at the seminary, who clearly are not giving me very objective advice on what to do. I wish I had my family to talk to, but when I've tried to, they take this kind of, "I told you so" attitude.

Before concluding the interview, Michael's clinician asked him if they had missed anything and whether he had any questions. Michael was satisfied that he had painted a clear picture of his difficulties and did not have any questions about the assessment process. Michael and his clinician then set a time for his feedback session, and Michael was invited to call if he had any questions or concerns in the interim.

Chapter 4

■ ■ ■

CONCEPTUALIZING THE CASE AND PLANNING TREATMENT

The clinician and client have now spent a few hours together. Plenty of information has been gathered—not only through the clinical interview, but also through other sources, including self-report measures and conversations with other professionals. Data were also obtained through observation of the client's behavior throughout the assessment process. The next step in this process is to spend some time figuring out how all this information comes together as a coherent whole. More specifically: How can the client's symptoms, and their etiological and maintaining variables, be best explained?

CONCEPTUALIZING THE CASE

As we noted in Chapter 1, case conceptualization is one of the most important skills that any clinician will learn. Through conceptualizing a case, a clinician develops a working hypothesis on how the client's particular problems can be understood in terms of the cognitive-behavioral model. This understanding then guides the process of treatment; in fact, Persons (1989) has referred to the case formulation as "the clinician's compass" (p. 37) for this reason.

Persons suggests that psychological problems occur at two levels: overt difficulties and underlying psychological mechanisms. Overt difficulties are the client's stated problems, like restrictive eating or depression or marital problems. Such problems can be described in terms of beliefs, behaviors, and emotions, in keeping with the cognitive model. The ways in which the problems are manifested across these three components are illustrative of the dysfunctionality of the underlying mechanism. Underlying psychological mechanisms, in other words, are "psychological deficits that underlie and cause the overt difficulties" (Persons, 1989, p. 1). Persons explains that the "underlying mechanisms can often be expressed in terms of one (or a few) irrational beliefs about the self" (p. 1), typically phrased in "If-then" statements. For example, if a patient holds the belief, "If I am fat, then no one will love me," this might manifest itself in dieting and excessive exercise, as well as dysfunctional thoughts and emotional reactiveness to eating, weight, and shape-related cues (the client's overt difficulties). This example demonstrates how the underlying mechanism can cause overt problems, but overt problems also serve to support underlying mechanisms. Following with this example, clients with eating problems often become quite socially isolated. Eating in front of others can be difficult, and both depression (which is often associated with eating problems) and the time-consuming nature of eating disorders can limit other social interactions as well. Social isolation (an overt problem) feeds back into the clients' belief that they are unlovable and that it must be because they are fat.

How does a clinician identify the mechanisms that underlie a client's overt difficulties? Persons's approach articulates this process through six steps (which we have summarized in Table 4.1) that not only help the clinician to determine this mechanism, but also to consider how the mechanism might impact on treatment. Persons suggests starting with a complete list of the client's obvious problems (Step 1) and then reasoning inductively toward a single underlying dysfunctional or core belief that could explain all the problems (Step 2). Then the therapist moves to con-

---

TABLE 4.1. Persons's Six-Step Case Conceptualization Model

1. Create an all-inclusive problem list that includes major symptoms and problems in functioning.

2. Propose an underlying mechanism (usually an irrational belief) that might underlie all the listed problems. To accomplish this, clinicians can ask themselves:
   a. What do all of these problems have in common?
   b. What belief would a person have who is behaving this way?
   c. What are the antecedents and consequences of the behavior?

3. Hypothesize how the underlying mechanism might produce the problems listed.

4. Explore the precipitants for the current problems. Does the proposed underlying mechanism match with the precipitants of the current problem?

5. Look for the origin of the mechanism (belief) in the client's early life.

6. Predict obstacles to treatment based on the formulation.

sider how the specific belief leads to the specific emotional, behavioral, and physiological symptoms and how those symptoms are maintained (Step 3). The clinician then essentially "tests" the hypothesis that this core belief underlies the client's current problems by considering whether the antecedents to the current problem are meaningfully related to the core belief (Step 4). The clinician also considers the possible origins of the central problem, usually by considering the learning experiences that the client had when growing up (typically via parents) which might have contributed to his or her current dysfunctional beliefs (Step 5). Finally, the clinician considers predicted obstacles to treatment stemming from the client's core beliefs (Step 6). Here are Persons's six steps in more detail.

1. The Problem List

As introduced in Chapter 3, a preliminary problem list is created at the end of the assessment session. The problem list should include the client's main presenting problems as well as other life issues and should be based on all of the sources of assessment information. The therapist then reviews this list, asking how these seemingly disparate problems might fit together within a cognitive-behavioral model.

At the end of Michael's assessment, he and his clinician created such a problem list. The obvious candidates were social anxiety, confusion about career choices, and family conflict. During Michael's assessment, his clinician sensed that he was experiencing some conflict about giving up the opportunity to have his own family should he enter the priesthood. Michael had not identified this as a problem, but Persons suggests that clinicians query clients about things that they observe during the assessment that might fit on the problem list. Michael's clinician did so, and they agreed to add it to the list and decide later in the course of therapy whether or not to deal with it.

2. The Proposed Underlying Mechanism

The goal here is to develop at least one possible explanation for all of the seemingly disparate problems with which the client presents. Based on cognitive-behavioral theory, the hypothesized mechanism is meant to serve an integrative function for all of the problems on the list. Persons has suggested that this integration often comes in the form of a central irrational belief. Any learned links among dysfunctional emotions, behaviors, and beliefs can be targeted for treatment, but the therapist must first understand which specific dysfunctional emotions and behaviors are linked with which specific dysfunctional beliefs.

Michael's clinician examined each of his problems in an attempt to come up with an underlying mechanism that would explain them all. She paid particular attention to the way that Michael thought about situations, as well as to the emotional, behavioral, and physiological responses that result from these interpretations.

Social Anxiety

The situational antecedent for Michael's main problem, social anxiety, was doing things in the presence of other people. The most problematic situation for Michael was public speaking, but even more casual social interactions were difficult. When he was in these situations, Michael worried that he would look anxious in front of other people and that they would associate these visible signs of anxiety with incompetence (*automatic thoughts*). In general, Michael held the *belief* that it was important to come across perfectly and that people who don't put forth a "perfect" impression were rejected by others. Given these thoughts, it was not surprising to learn that Michael typically reacted with anxiety (*emotional response*) to being in social situations, or even to the prospect of being in them. Concomitant with this emotional response, Michael experienced *physiological changes*, including blushing, shaking, and sweating that made him feel ever more certain that everyone could see these symptoms and would draw the conclusion that he was anxious and incompetent (*automatic thoughts*). In the past, Michael's concerns about social interactions had led to a great deal of avoidance (*behavioral response*). Michael explained that this was driven by the *belief*, "If I couldn't come across perfectly to others, I thought it wasn't even worth trying." Since entering the seminary, avoidance had become more difficult. Michael had started to engage in other behaviors to try to control his anxiety and ensure that people would not see it. He engaged primarily in overpreparation (*behavioral response*). He would stay up late at night studying so that if he was called on in class, he could be sure to answer questions correctly. He also practiced sermons and readings numerous times before church services. Typically, Michael did succeed at answering questions correctly, and delivered thoughtful, well-spoken sermons. He attributed this "success" to his overpreparation. In other words, his behaviors fed back into his beliefs—Michael believed that he was more prone to making mistakes than others and, therefore, that he had to work extra hard to prevent this most feared outcome (*beliefs*). Since he never did "mess up," Michael continued to hold the belief that if he did, he would be rejected by others.

Career Choice

Michael's recent decision to take a leave of absence from medicine and explore his religious calling spurred his current difficulties around his career choice (*event*). Now at the seminary, Michael was having doubts about whether he made the right decision. He explained during his assessment, "If I leave, people are going to know that I couldn't hack it" (*belief*). He also stated, "You'd think at my age, I could make the right decision about something as important as this" (*belief*). These kinds of beliefs made Michael feel very anxious, were associated with a great deal of physiological reactivity, and generally led him to continually put off thinking about his career choice (*behavioral response*). During his assessment, Michael alluded to fear of rejection in this area, too. He explained that if he left medicine, his friends and colleagues in medicine would no longer want to associate with him and that if he left the seminary, his classmates and superiors there similarly would not want to associate with him. It was clear to his clinician that it was not his choice per se that Michael believed would lead to rejection, but rather his inability to make the "right" decision about his career and stick with it.

Family Conflict

Michael's family conflict was also clearly tied to his career choices. His parents had been proud of his career in medicine and, despite their own faith, they were not particularly pleased with his consideration of the priesthood (*event*). When Michael talked about his family's reaction to his decision, he explained, "They didn't want me to do this, and it's going to be really embarrassing if they end up being right"(*emotion*). Again, Michael had got himself into a situation where it was impossible for him to "win." If he stayed in the priesthood, he assumed his family would think he made a huge mistake and therefore would reject him. Yet he also believed that if he left and returned to medicine, his family would still think he made a big mistake by even considering the priesthood and that this too could lead to rejection. Worrying so much about his family's reactions to his career choice had recently been leading to some avoidance on Michael's part (*behavioral response*). In the month leading up to his evaluation, Michael had missed a number of family events and had been calling his family members less frequently, simply to avoid having to talk about these difficult issues and hear about his family's disappointment with him.

Decisions about Family

This was the issue Michael was most reluctant to discuss. Since this response to the clinician's questioning was so different from Michael's responses to other lines of questioning, this behavior was quite notable. Michael told the clinician that he had always thought he would get married and have a family, but that he completely accepted that as a priest, he would be fully committed to God and to his faith. However, his reluctance to talk further suggested to the clinician that his thoughts about this difficult issue might be more complicated than Michael was letting on.

How does a clinician take all of this information and put it together to arrive at a cohesive underlying mechanism to explain the client's problems? Persons suggests that the clinician consider *the way that the client describes the chief complaint*. Recall that when Michael first called to set up his appointment, he said, "Well, I know it sounds dumb for a grown man, but I've been having a lot of problems with speaking up in public. I just went back to school and can't speak up in class and the work I am doing now requires a lot of public speaking that also makes me feel uncomfortable. I'm always screwing up—it's just terrible." Right from the start, Michael talked about having very high standards for himself and believing not only that "screwing up" was a bad thing, but also that even *being* anxious was unacceptable for a person of his age. Given that he was even concerned about what the clinician thought of him in their initial interaction ("I know it sounds dumb for a grown man . . ."), it was reasonable to wonder whether Michael's concerns extended beyond disappointing himself to also disappointing others and suffering the resulting consequences.

Perhaps the most helpful way to arrive at the underlying mechanism is to examine the problem list and ask: "*What do all these problems have in common?*" (Persons, 1989, p. 51). For items on the list that are behavioral in nature (e.g., avoiding public speaking), clinicians can ask themselves, "What belief would a person who is behaving like this have?" When Michael was describing his concerns about public speaking, he reported the following automatic thoughts: "I always look anxious" and "Everyone notices how anxious I am" as well as "They all think I'm an idiot" and "I can never get it quite right." The clinician should help the client to go beyond these thoughts and consider what would be the ultimate consequence if these thoughts were indeed "accurate." What would be the consequence for Michael of people noticing his anxiety and thinking that he was an "idiot"? Michael believed that if people made these interpretations, he would be rejected by his peers, his superiors and his parishioners. He also believed that if he made an "incorrect" choice in life, he would be rejected by colleagues, friends, and even his family members. It seemed like Michael had set up for himself a life where he feared rejection by someone regardless of how he behaved or what choices he made. Michael's clinician therefore concluded that the central core belief that seemed to underlie Michael's problems was "I am bound to be rejected."

3. How the Proposed Mechanism Produces the Problems Listed

The next step (and perhaps the most important one) in the case formulation is stating how the hypothesized central problem leads to all of the problems on the list. As we have just noted, Michael seemed to have a great fear of rejection. He believed he was more prone to making mistakes than others, believed that people reject others for making mistake, and, not surprisingly, believed that he should avoid making mistakes at all costs.

Michael's overt problems "made sense" when viewed as consequences of his core underlying beliefs. Whenever possible he avoided social situations completely, because this protected him from the possibility of making mistakes and being rejected. When he did have to enter social situations, he overprepared and carefully measured everything he said to make sure he didn't make a mistake. He also seemed to have difficulty making decisions about his path in life, and discussing such decisions with people he was close to, for fear that he would make the wrong decision, be a disappointment, and ultimately be rejected. Figure 4.1 shows how Michael's case fits into a cognitive-behavioral model.

4. Precipitants of the Current Problems

In this stage of the case conceptualization, the clinician considers whether the hypothesized mechanism (the central irrational belief) is meaningfully related to the antecedents of the client's current problems. In effect, this attempt to match up mechanism with precipitant serves as a test of the proposed mechanism. If Michael's core belief was "I am bound to be rejected," then it would be expected that the precipitant of his current problems would be an event or situation that brought up these concerns for him.

This was most certainly the case. Remember that Michael had always been socially anxious, but he had waited until age 40 to come to treatment. It was quite clear to Michael's clinician that there had been a number of events recently in which Michael worried that people would perceive that he made a mistake, judge him negatively for doing so, and ultimately reject him. His parents thought that his desire to enter the priesthood was a mistake. If he decided to pursue it, Michael thought it possible that they might distance themselves from him. If he decided to return to his job in medicine, his fellow seminarians would reject him. A complicating factor for Michael was also his perception of God. Michael felt that he had been called to the priesthood and worried that if he ignored that calling, God might reject him as well.

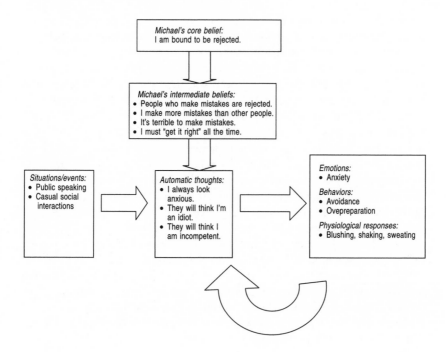

FIGURE 4.1. Applying the cognitive model to Michael's underlying core belief. Adapted from J. S. Beck (1995, p. 18). Copyright 1995 by The Guilford Press. Adapted by permission.

5. Origin of the Mechanism in the Client's Early Life

In the preceding paragraph, we discussed events that had happened to Michael recently that would support the hypothesized mechanism for his difficulties. Michael's belief that he might be rejected also suggests that he had experiences when he was growing up that contributed to this concern. Persons recommends looking further back into the client's personal history to see if there is additional evidence in support of this hypothesis. This recommendation might seem surprising to beginning clinicians, since one of the unique aspects of CBT is its focus on the present (as is further outlined later in this chapter). While it is certainly true that CBT clinicians are *primarily* interested in the individual's present behavior, having a historical record of an individual's life and his or her experiences may help to explain how problem behaviors developed in the first place. This knowledge can then help the clinician understand the factors that maintain maladaptive thoughts and behaviors in the present and tailor therapy to "chip away" at these maintaining factors. It is worth noting that sharing this information likely makes clients feel more understood, which can certainly strengthen the therapeutic relationship.

During the administration of the social phobia section of the SCID, Michael was asked when he first started to have difficulties with social anxiety. He reported that he had been socially anxious for as long as he could remember, and he posited that this was due to growing up in a home with highly critical parents. He said that when he was a child, his mother would kick him under the table if he said something of which she did not approve. Before going out to social events, his mother would tell him to try not to blush so much. He recalled a few occasions when she was standing across a room from him and pointed to her own face if she saw his becoming very red. Later, Michael's mother would tell him that his blushing would make other people think he was a "nervous Nellie" and that "no one wants to be friends with a nervous Nellie."

As soon as Michael enrolled in school, it was clear that he was very bright. Nevertheless, this became another arena fraught with potential rejection. His teachers expected a great deal of him, so if he did have a hard time with something (or even worse, made a careless mistake), this often elicited lectures from teachers about "not reaching his potential." He attended a private school with high academic standards, and reenrollment each year was contingent on excellent grades. Each year Michael lived with the fear that he would be asked to leave.

He explained that this had been less of a concern in the past few years as he headed up the pathology lab where he worked and was not really checked on by colleagues. Yet, as already noted, this concern about making mistakes reemerged when he entered the seminary. Michael explained that excellence was expected of all students and that not knowing the correct answer to a question in class could result in a lecture about motivation to pursue this very challenging, difficult, and special path in life. Furthermore, continued evidence of "failure" would of course result in a student being told that this special path was not for him.

6. Predicted Obstacles to Treatment Based on the Formulation

Persons has recommended carefully examining the proposed mechanism for the client's problems and considering the role that it might play in treatment. For Michael, concern about being rejected could certainly affect the course of treatment. For Michael, rejection came about when anything was done less than perfectly. Michael's clinician knew that she needed to be aware of the way in which he tackled homework assignments early in treatment. Some clients who are very concerned about making mistakes avoid doing homework for fear that they will be judged negatively if they do not do it perfectly. Others will do their homework but will spend excessive time making sure that they write neatly, spell everything correctly, and explain things "just so." Clients like this will often seek reassurance from clinicians, checking to make sure that they have completed the assignment the way that the clinician wants it to be completed. Michael's clinician was mindful of setting the tone early in therapy that homework did not have to be completed perfectly and would not be a basis of evaluation. There was also some concern that Michael might avoid talking about issues that were very difficult for him for fear that the clinician would become one more person in his life who would judge him negatively for the choices he had made. Most notable was his confusion about having a family. It was possible that Michael was reluctant to discuss this for fear that the clinician would judge him negatively for choosing to give this opportunity up for his faith.

HOW DOES THE CASE CONCEPTUALIZATION INFORM THE TREATMENT PLAN?

Devising the case conceptualization naturally leads to the evolution of a plan for treatment. While the idea that the case conceptualization informs the treatment plan becomes routine to seasoned clinicians, beginners should put a detailed treatment plan in writing and discuss it with their supervisors. Articulating the plan in this way (rather than just having a version of it in your mind) ensures that clinicians have a sense of how a case is going to unfold from start to finish. This does not mean that modifications are not permitted. However, when modifications are made, they should be based on the ongoing reformulation of the case conceptualization.

What Was the Treatment Plan for Michael?

Let's consider how the conceptualization of Michael's case informed his treatment plan. Michael was concerned that others would reject him if he were to make mistakes. He further believed that making mistakes was a highly likely outcome for him; this was not surprising, given the excessively high standards he set for himself, and his belief that making mistakes came at a significant cost (rejection). These beliefs contributed to Michael's significant social anxiety, and the concomitants of it—namely, avoidance and the use of all sorts of safety behaviors (like overpreparation) when he could not avoid a situation outright. These behavioral responses prevented Michael from learning that his beliefs about mistakes were inaccurate and exaggerated, and that the consequences of making mistakes were far less dire than Michael predicted. At the same time, when dire predictions about mistakes and rejection did not occur, Michael credited his avoidance or safety behaviors, thus reinforcing those behaviors.

This led Michael's clinician to conclude that treatment should be focused on helping Michael explore his beliefs about making mistakes and about being rejected by others. How could CBT be used to accomplish this goal? Michael could be helped to directly challenge his dysfunctional beliefs through cognitive restructuring. Behaviorally, Michael would also have to stop avoiding feared social situations as well as to do away with the overpreparation that he relied on when he could not avoid them. These behavioral changes would allow Michael to further test his beliefs that he was particularly prone to making mistakes and that mistakes would lead others to reject him. They would also enable him to explore his beliefs about looking anxious, which he believed was perceived by others in much the same way as forgetting a word or having a long pause in a conversation. Michael assumed that all of these "mistakes" were just variations on ways that he would be perceived as incompetent, and then rejected, by people around him. These intentional changes in belief and behavior would likely result in Michael learning that (1) he was not more likely to make mistakes than others and (2) when he did make mistakes, the consequences were not dire. In fact, he would likely learn that most people wouldn't notice his mistakes at all, and that when they did, it was very unlikely that such occurrences would lead to rejection. Figure 4.2 illustrates a cognitive-behavioral model for understanding the maintenance and treatment of Michael's social phobia.

What about Michael's other problems? Once he learned that he rarely made mistakes and that when he did make them, the result was not rejection, would his other problems be resolved as well? This was certainly possible, but at the very least, the lessons Michael learned when working on social anxiety would likely help him to better work through these other problems either with the help of a therapist, or on his own. Nevertheless, his therapist was aware that these other problems could interfere with the treatment focused on social phobia or be left unresolved at the end of it. In these cases, cognitive and behavioral techniques could be employed in a more flexible manner to deal with Michael's concerns about work, his familial relationships, and the prospect of having his own family in the future. At this point in treatment planning, a specific plan was not devised for dealing with these other problems. Rather, the clinician kept in mind that treatment might not end after a time-limited course of CBT for social phobia. As treatment progressed, Michael's clinician knew that she would have to continuously revise her conceptualization of Michael's case and their plan for treatment depending on how some of these other issues evolved.

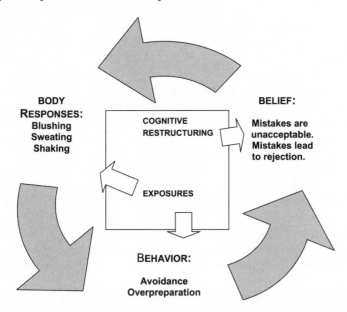

FIGURE 4.2. A cognitive-behavioral model of how Michael's anxiety is maintained and techniques to treat it.

TWO FINAL POINTS ON TREATMENT PLANNING

Once the case has been conceptualized, beginning clinicians often have two questions: (1) How do I decide how to structure treatment? and (2) If the client has more than one problem, how do I decide where to begin? In the remainder of this chapter, we discuss these two dilemmas.

A Guide for the Treatment: Using Treatment Manuals

With the goal of treatment defined and a rough idea of what must occur in therapy to help clients meet these goals, the next question is how to devise a structure for the therapy. An excellent option, particularly for beginning clinicians, is to use a treatment manual. Treatment manuals provide structure to a case, giving clinicians a clear sense of how therapy should unfold to help clients work through a specific problem (e.g., depression, body image problems, etc.). Manuals help alleviate the anxiety that beginning clinicians experience with respect to knowing what to say and do in therapy sessions, freeing up attention to focus on the client.

Therapy manuals typically include some information on the nature of the problem that is the focus of treatment, explain how treatment should proceed, include helpful forms and handouts, and sometimes even include tips for dealing with difficult issues in therapy, like noncompliance. Although manuals outline a standard treatment protocol, therapy with each client will be unique. As such, it is important for clinicians to use the case conceptualization to consider how therapy will likely unfold with each client. Clinicians should consider what kinds of beliefs will likely be the focus of cognitive work and what sort of behavioral interventions will be useful. These specific ideas for treatment should all be geared at helping clients with their overt difficulties, as well as with the core dysfunctional beliefs underlying these difficulties. Clinicians should also consider whether the case conceptualization gives us any clues to foreseeable roadblocks in carrying out the treatment. For example, a client who is very distrustful of others might be skeptical of CBT and of the clinician, particularly early on in treatment. Being mindful of this will allow the clinician to be prepared and give some thought to how to work with the client if he or she in fact exhibits this kind of distrust.

Michael's clinician decided to use a specific treatment manual to guide his treatment—specifically, a social phobia treatment manual by Debra Hope and colleagues (Hope, Heimberg, Juster, & Turk, 2000). The manual includes psychoeducational material, as well as guidance on how to do cognitive restructuring and carry out behavioral exposures. At the end of Michael's feedback session, his therapist reviewed the treatment manual and mapped out a treatment plan based on it, with specifically defined treatment goals. This treatment plan is shown in Table 4.2. Michael's clinician also gave some thought to potential roadblocks to treatment. The case conceptualization has already alerted the clinician that Michael's concern over making mistakes and being rejected might affect how he engaged in the treatment and carried out homework (e.g., spending too much time on homework to make it perfect). Similarly, she recognized that treatment could be used as a venue for Michael to practice being less precise and careful with his work (e.g., asking him to intentionally do a less than perfect job with homework).

Which Problem(s) Should Be Treated First?

Beginning clinicians often have a problem figuring out "where to start" with clients who have multiple presenting complaints. It would be terribly confusing (for both clinician and client) to try to deal with everything at once—and it would likely lead to little progress in any one area. Following a case formulation approach like that espoused by Persons can be a great help in this respect. The problem list that at first seems so disjointed becomes unified by the proposed underlying mechanism. Un-

TABLE 4.2. Michael's Treatment Plan

- Proposed length of treatment: 16–20 sessions (once weekly, 1-hour sessions).
- Will use Hope et al. (2000) treatment manual for social anxiety.
- Main treatment goal: To help Michael challenge his beliefs about the probability and cost of making mistakes, and about the fear of being rejected if he does make mistakes.

Proposed outline and goals for treatment

Session 1: Educational material on social anxiety

Goals: To normalize the experience of social anxiety; to introduce Michael to the cognitive-behavioral model for understanding and treating social anxiety; to set the stage for a collaborative treatment process where Michael would learn to become his own therapist.

Session 2: Finish educational material, design hierarchy of feared situations

Goals: See Session 1. Identify feared and avoided social situations, make a plan for how exposure to these situations will proceed.

Session 3: Introduce cognitive restructuring (CR)

Goals: To introduce Michael to the idea that our interpretation of situations are problematic—not the situations themselves; to teach Michael how to identify, challenge, and reframe dysfunctional thoughts.

Session 4: Continue CR, plan first exposure to low-hierarchy item

Goals: To continue skill building (in relation to the cognitive restructuring); to introduce Michael to the idea of using behavioral exposures to further challenge dysfunctional beliefs; to teach Michael how to set up a behavioral exposure.

Session 5: Carry out first exposure

Goals: To demonstrate to Michael how exposure to feared situations can result in new learning as existing dysfunctional beliefs are challenged.

Sessions 6–18: Exposures and continuing CR and examination of core beliefs (with flexibility for dealing with related issues)

Goals: To continue using cognitive and behavioral strategies to challenge dysfunctional beliefs and change problematic behaviors; to help Michael internalize these new beliefs and behaviors and generalize them to situations that have not been specifically confronted in therapy; to help Michael use cognitive and behavioral strategies to work on some of the other problems in his life.

Sessions 19 and 20: Relapse prevention, goal setting, termination

Goals: To prepare Michael for termination of therapy; to help Michael have realistic expectations for the future; to work with Michael to create goals to continue working on when therapy is over; to help Michael feel comfortable with termination by reflecting on what he has learned and on his newfound ability to be his own therapist.

derstanding this mechanism serves as a compass for treatment, providing direction and structure for the therapy process.

When working in settings where *disorders* are treated, this issue can become a bit trickier. One way to address this issue is to simply ask clients which problem is the most distressing to them. What can be even more helpful, particularly with complex cases, is to spend some time discussing with clients the functional relationship between their various disorders. Some difficulties may seem to have no meaningful relationship at all. If a client presents with fear of snakes and marital problems, it is unlikely (but not impossible) that the two are meaningfully related. Some disorders are related, but it seems reasonable to expect that one disorder might remit with treatment for the other disorder. For example, a client with comorbid OCD and depression might believe that if she was no longer having numerous intrusive thoughts and spending much of her day carrying out compulsions, she would no longer feel depressed. In such a case, it would be appropriate to focus on the OCD and only attend separately to the depression if it interferes with treatment or remains a problem once the OCD has been successfully treated.

In other cases, it might be essential to work on one disorder, in order to ready the person for working on the other disorder(s). For example, another client with comorbid OCD and depression might tell you that she feels so depressed that she is having difficulties going about basic tasks of daily living, like showering and eating proper meals. It would be very difficult for such a client to engage in an active treatment like CBT for OCD. It would be best to work on the depression first, and once the client felt more energetic and motivated, shift to working on the OCD.

From time to time, a client's perception of the most significant problem will be inconsistent with the clinician's perception. In that situation, it is reasonable to express your surprise to the client. Consider a client with panic attacks, bulimia, and depression:

CLINICIAN: So, you consider the panic attacks your biggest problem right now?

CLIENT: Yeah, for sure.

CLINICIAN: Hmmmm. That surprises me a bit. During our assessment, you told me that you have panic attacks pretty infrequently.

CLIENT: Yeah, I do. But they're pretty awful when they come on.

CLINICIAN: So, when they do happen, they get you pretty stressed out and kind of foul up your day?

CLIENT: Yeah. They definitely stress me out. I don't know about fouling up a whole day, though. They don't last that long you know.

CLINICIAN: How about the problems with your eating? Can they foul up a whole day?

CLIENT: They foul up every day. I already told you—I'm bingeing like three times a day. And then I throw up. And I feel so gross that I have to have a shower to get cleaned up and calm down. It's awful. I've missed five classes in the past week.

CLINICIAN: So, it sounds like the bulimia might be interfering more than the panic attacks.

CLIENT: I guess.

CLINICIAN: It sounds like you might be feeling like working on the eating is a bit more stressful right now than working on the panic.

CLIENT: Well, obviously.

CLINICIAN: It can be very hard, I agree. Is it worth giving it a try for a few weeks and seeing how it goes?

CLIENT: I guess.

To summarize, a lack of congruence between the clinician's clinical judgment and the client's judgment warrants examination. Sometimes clients avoid working on the problem that they perceive as most difficult to treat or that they have some ambivalence about working on.

In Michael's case, both Michael and his clinician were in agreement that they should focus on social phobia first. Michael had other problems (career choice, family conflict, decisions about family) that would not be the initial focus of treatment, but which would likely come up from time to time. While the social phobia treatment manual offers no specific guidance on these possibly related issues, they would be dealt with as they arose, using the same cognitive-behavioral techniques that were being used to help Michael work on his social anxiety. In other words, the manual includes treatment techniques that are broadly applicable.

Michael's therapist would have to continuously revisit their decision to focus first on his social phobia. While it is perfectly fine to dedicate brief amounts of time to his related issues as they came up, the treatment plan would have to be revisited if one of these related problems became so salient that it got in the way of treatment for social phobia. A more likely outcome, however, is that these related difficulties would gradually improve as Michael continues treatment for social phobia. After all, if the case conceptualization was correct, and the underlying core belief was accurately identified, treatment directed toward this belief (e.g., treatment for social phobia) should also bring improvement to Michael's other problems. As Michael came to see that he was unlikely to make mistakes, and that mistakes were not necessarily associated with rejection, it was expected that he would be more able to come to other decisions in his life without being clouded by these fears.

To summarize, it is important to always remember that case conceptualization is an ongoing process. Although clinicians should start treatment with a plan for how it should proceed, they must evaluate the status of the case on an ongoing basis and decide if they should deviate from the initial plan to best meet the needs of the client. This process will be demonstrated throughout the next few chapters as the case of Michael unfolds.

Chapter 5

■ ■ ■

GIVING FEEDBACK TO CLIENTS AND WRITING THE ASSESSMENT REPORT

Upon completing an assessment, experienced clinicians often give the client feedback immediately. This is usually not the case with trainees. Most sites expect trainees to discuss assessments with their supervisors and have some help in establishing the diagnosis and formulating the case. Furthermore, some states and provinces actually forbid non-licensed clinicians from communicating diagnoses to clients. Trainees should be sure they understand the laws in their particular jurisdiction.

When considering how much information to give clients, the basic rule of thumb is to keep it simple. Providing clients with too much information, or information that is too complex, can be overwhelming and can result in their coming away from the session feeling confused. The client's understanding is important not only to the success of the treatment, but also because the process of obtaining the client's informed consent to treatment is embedded in the feedback process. The main tasks of a feedback session are (1) to review the client's strengths; (2) to review the client's problems (problem list) and explain the diagnosis that fits those problems; (3) to share and discuss the case conceptualization; and (4) to review the treatment options with their advantages and disadvantages, and recommend treatment. A summary of tips for giving feedback is included in Table 5.1.

REVIEWING THE CLIENT'S STRENGTHS

Feedback can be made more positive by pointing out clients' strengths. We are often so focused on letting clients know what their problems are

TABLE 5.1. Tips for the Feedback Process
___

1. Always be mindful of the client's reactions to the feedback. Help the client to process difficult information.

2. Point out the client's strengths, rather than just discussing weakness and problems.

3. Propose the problem list, diagnosis, and case conceptualization.
   - When discussing the problem list . . .
     - Make sure nothing was left off.
     - Ensure the client that the list should err on the side of inclusiveness—the list does not necessarily mean that he or she *must* deal with each of these problems.
   - When discussing the diagnosis . . .
     - Review the client's symptoms that led you to arrive at this decision.
     - Explain the cognitive-behavioral model for understanding the maintenance of these symptoms.
   - When discussing the case conceptualization . . .
     - Check that it fits with the client's view of his or her problems.
     - Revise the conceptualization in light of the client's feedback.

4. Explain treatment options.
   - Review how CBT could help the client's specific problems.
   - Outline other treatment options.
   - Discuss the benefits and drawbacks of all options presented.

5. Make your treatment recommendations.

6. Make it clear that questions are welcome.
___

and what they need to do to improve their functioning that we forget to also emphasize their strengths. Some clients who have very severe problems still manage to function quite well in at least some areas of their lives. Other clients are very good at seeking out the help that they need, either by seeking support from significant others or by making the effort to learn more about their difficulties and how to treat them. Certainly, seeking treatment is, in and of itself, a strength. During the feedback process, clients should be reminded of these positive qualities. In general, feedback should be given in an empathic, positive, and hopeful way. Starting with strengths helps set this tone.

REVIEWING THE PROBLEM LIST AND DIAGNOSES

The second step in providing feedback is to review the problem list with the client and ensure that no items are missing. Remind clients that they will not necessarily work on all of the listed problems during therapy, but it is better to be all-inclusive at this time. The various assessment tools will have identified the specific behavioral, cognitive, and emotional aspects of the main problems. These key symptoms can also be briefly outlined.

As in Michael's case, the problem list might also include specific psychiatric diagnoses. When this is the case, clinicians should also share with the client any diagnoses that have been made, explaining how these diagnostic decisions were arrived at. In other words, the therapist should point out the client's specific symptoms that lead to the specific diagnoses. Most notably, the clinician should also explain to the client (in cognitive-behavioral terms) why his or her problems have been maintained over time even though the client might have tried quite hard to make changes alone.

It is important for novice clinicians to consider how clients may react to receiving a diagnosis and be prepared to process these reactions with them. Some clients associate mental illness with stigma and might be resistant to the idea of having a mental disorder. Other clients might accept that they have a diagnosis but might see it as a mark of weakness or as an indication that they are in some way flawed. Similarly, some clients will react with feelings of hopelessness, perceiving their diagnosis as beyond their control and therefore, unchangeable. Many clients, however, have quite a positive reaction to having a name for their difficulties. They might have spent years feeling different and alone. Knowing that their difficulties have a name and that many other people have the same problems can be a source of great relief.

SHARING THE CASE CONCEPTUALIZATION

With the problem list articulated, the clinician can now share with the client his or her conceptualization of the case—in other words, how these seemingly disparate problems might fit together and how this integrated perspective will inform treatment. It is important that the client understands the case conceptualization and sees it as fitting his or her situation. Although you are the expert at assessing patients, conceptualizing cases, and coming up with a treatment plan, clients are the experts in the difficulties that they have experienced. Clients can be asked, "Does this match how you see the problems?" If they see the conceptualization as "off base," clinicians should be open to feedback and to making appropriate changes, being mindful that case conceptualization is an ongoing process.

REVIEWING TREATMENT OPTIONS

With the core problems defined, and a unifying underlying mechanism proposed, the clinician can then present treatment options to clients. Various options should be presented (e.g., CBT, other forms of psychotherapy, medication) and the advantages and disadvantages of each outlined. Throughout, it is important to ask the client if he or she may have misunderstood or missed anything important. Be mindful that clients can sometimes express confusion or uncertainly through their body language. If a client looks confused, it is perfectly appropriate to pause and say, "Do you have any questions at this point?" or "Is there anything I can do to make all of this clearer?" Through your own behavior, make it clear to clients that it is appropriate and, in fact, beneficial, for them to ask questions.

Helping Clients to Make an Informed Decision about CBT

If you believe that CBT is the right approach for the client (or would be an important component of a broader treatment program—one that includes medication, for example), your next job is to help clients make an informed decision about whether or not they will pursue this treatment. Although CBT might seem like a very sensible approach to those who use it every day, most clients are unfamiliar with it. In presenting treatment options to clients, it is important to explain the cognitive-behavioral approach and give clients all of the information they need to make an educated decision about whether it is right for them.

When this feedback typically occurs depends on the clinic in which you work. In the case of Michael, treatment options were discussed during a separate feedback session that occurred following the assessment. If a feedback session does not occur, treatment options can be discussed at the end of the assessment. Obviously, some clients will want to learn about treatment options even before they are assessed for treatment. This is fine, so long as you are clear that treatment recommendations are best made once the assessment is complete. In these situations, treatment can be discussed in a general way and then, following the assessment, the discussion can be made specific to the client's individual concerns.

It is helpful to provide clients with a "snapshot" of what CBT looks like. Keep in mind that clients sometimes do not know what the word "cognitive" means. Explain that when we talk about cognitions, we are simply talking about thoughts, and that CBT is focused on helping clients to change the thoughts that they have in particular situations so that they will begin to view the world in a more accurate and adaptive way. Give examples that are relevant to clients to help them to understand this process.

In briefly explaining the behavioral aspect of treatment to our clients, we can explain to them that it can be hard to simply change our thoughts. Clients can tell clinicians whatever they think we want to hear, but to make truly meaningful and enduring changes in the way that they view the world, clients need to have new experiences. In CBT, clients are asked to try out behaviors that are entirely new to them or that they have not engaged in for a long time, and, often, they are asked to cease dysfunctional or unhealthy behaviors. In explaining these changes, again draw on examples that are relevant to clients' experiences.

It is important to describe to clients what CBT is all about and to illuminate what is unique about it. There are four essential points to share. First, clients should be told about the stance taken in CBT—one of collaborative empiricism, where clinician and client are partners in treating the client's difficulties. Second, clients should know that CBT is a time-limited treatment. On this note, clients should be told how it is that goals can be accomplished so rapidly in CBT—namely, that CBT is an active, problem-focused, and present-focused approach to treating psychological problems. Finally, clients should be told that cognitive-behavioral clinicians are scientifically inclined and emphasize use of techniques that have been proven effective.

The Stance of Collaborative Empiricism

In our experience, the aspect of CBT that most surprises clients is the stance of *collaborative empiricism* that is taken by the clinician and the client. Their image of therapy often involves an individual free associating, waiting for the "all-knowing" clinician to provide an interpretation of the origins of the client's difficulties.

The stance of collaborative empiricism is perhaps best exhibited when the clinician uses the technique of Socratic questioning. In analytic therapies, it is most often the case that the clinician makes interpretative statements; in CBT, we ask questions, leading clients to their own interpretations of thoughts and behaviors. This is not to say that we do not have an idea of what we want the client to think about particular issues. For example, if a depressed client says, "Things will never change for me," our inclination (and likely what we would do when speaking to friends or family members) would be to say "But of course things will change for you." According to J. S. Beck (1995), making this kind of statement can come across as an effort to "persuade" the client of the "clinician's viewpoint" (p. 8). The harm in using persuasion is twofold. First, it can communicate to clients that their thoughts or beliefs are "wrong." Second, by persuading clients to see the world in another way, we deprive them of the opportunity to learn valuable skills. Specifically, in CBT, we want to help clients "determine the accuracy and utility of [their] ideas via a careful review of data" (J. S. Beck, 1995, p. 8). Therefore, instead of telling the client that things will change for him or her, we could ask, "Do you have any evidence that things *might* change for you in the future?" or "Is there any other way that you could think about the future?" Using Socratic questioning communicates to clients that you would like to know what they think, that they can help you to understand their experiences and, in turn, you can guide them to come to their own solutions for a problem.

The Time-Limited Nature of CBT

New clients are also often surprised by the *time-limited* nature of CBT. Clients often have a vision of therapy lasting for years. In CBT, clinicians start a course of treatment having a sense of how long it will last and share this plan with their clients. This estimate of the duration of therapy is based on research and published therapy manuals, as well as experience with other clients. The client's unique presentation might also impact on the clinician's sense of how long the treatment might last. A client who is having moderately severe panic attacks and engaging in very minimal avoidance behavior might do quite well with six sessions of CBT. In contrast, a client who is having frequent and severe panic attacks and has been housebound for the past 2 years might need closer to 20 sessions of CBT. While there is no set rule for the duration of CBT, it seems that most problems can be treated quite effectively in 20 or fewer sessions.

CBT Is an Active, Problem-Focused, and Present-Focused Approach

Clients should also understand *how* significant gains can be made in CBT in a relatively short period of time. CBT is an efficient approach to treatment because it is *active, problem-focused, and present-focused.* Again, if we consider the mental image that people hold of therapy, it often involves clients spending years talking about their early experiences and trying to come to some insight on where their difficulties might have come from. In CBT, only minimal attention is paid to the origins of a problem, with focus being placed instead on changing current behaviors and thinking patterns in order to improve functioning.

Is CBT for Everyone?

Despite its broad applicability, CBT is not for every problem or for everyone. Therefore, when making treatment recommendations, clinicians should be open to the possibility that the client might be better suited to some other approach.

When might CBT be inappropriate? As we have noted, CBT is an active approach to treatment—both in terms of cognitions and behaviors. Clients with severe intellectual impairments are not well-suited to CBT that places a heavy emphasis on cognitive components of treatment (although behavior therapies are very beneficial to such clients). Similarly, clients in poor physical health might have difficulties with the demands of some CBT programs (e.g., exposure and ritual prevention treatment for persons with some subtypes of OCD, like hoarding; interoceptive exposure for clients with panic disorder). Other clients simply might not like the idea of CBT. They might prefer a less structured, supportive psychotherapy instead. While we should educate clients about what CBT entails and how it might help them, if they are not interested in pursuing it, we should provide them with appropriate referrals, rather than trying to convince them that CBT is for them.

Even if clients are clearly enthusiastic about CBT, it is our responsibility to also let them know about the "disadvantages" of treatments. CBT is time-consuming, requiring regular sessions with the clinician and commitment by the client to complete assignments between sessions. It can be costly, and therapy is not always covered by insurance. It requires that clients be willing to put themselves into difficult situations and make some pretty significant changes to both their belief system and the way that they live their lives. It is important that clients know this before making a decision.

Before addressing some commonly asked questions that can arise during the process of giving feedback, let's review the feedback that was given to Michael following his assessment.

MICHAEL'S FEEDBACK SESSION

Michael came back to the clinic about a week after his assessment. He warmly greeted the clinician, told her that he had found their meeting very informative and that he was looking forward to getting started with treatment. The clinician started off the session by pointing out Michael's strengths.

Reviewing Strengths

CLINICIAN: I am looking forward to our meeting today. I really enjoyed talking with you last week too. It was clear to me that you had given a lot of thought to the difficulties that you are having and you seem very motivated to make some positive changes in your life.

MICHAEL: Absolutely. I really need to do something about this social anxiety.

CLINICIAN: How was the past week for you?

MICHAEL: Brutal. I was up all night on Sunday preparing for class on Monday, and then I had to lead a service on Tuesday, so I was up for most of Monday night too. When I start the week like this, by the end of the week I am a basket case, and I think it's more because of sleep deprivation than because of social anxiety.

Reviewing the Problem List

CLINICIAN: I can see that. Well, let's start out by reviewing the problem list that we constructed last week. The first problem that we put on the list was your social anxiety. When we spoke about your social anxiety last week, we found that it had a number of characteristics. For example, you feel a great deal of distress in social situations, particularly when speaking in front of others and, to a lesser extent, when chatting more casually with people. Showing signs of anxiety, like blushing or sweating, greatly increases your fear and distress. To deal with the anxiety, you've tried to avoid social and public situations or, alternatively, put a lot of effort into making sure you don't come across badly when you can't avoid them. All of this avoidance and distress has negatively impacted your professional life and your personal life. Is this all correct?

MICHAEL: Yes. That sounds about right.

CLINICIAN: The pattern of anxiety I've just outlined fits with a diagnosis of social phobia. Social phobia is a disorder characterized by excessive concern about the way that other people judge or evaluate you. It's actually one of the most common psychological disorders, experienced by about 13% of Americans at some time in their lives.

MICHAEL: You're kidding. I had no idea it was so common.

CLINICIAN: Yes, it is.

MICHAEL: Wow, that makes me feel a bit better about things.

CLINICIAN: I'm glad to hear that. Do you have any questions about social phobia that I can answer?

MICHAEL: Not right now.

CLINICIAN: Okay. Just let me know if you think of any. For now, let's look at the rest of your problem list. We also noted problems with career choice, conflicts with your family over the possibility of you entering the priesthood, and issues related to deciding whether or not to have a family of your own. Over the week, did you think about any other problems you'd like to add to the list?

MICHAEL: Isn't that enough? (*laughing*) Seriously though, it seems fine.

CLINICIAN: Okay, so we agree that the problem list is complete?

MICHAEL: Sure.

Sharing the Case Conceptualization

CLINICIAN: Now, I'd like to review with you how I've come to make sense of the various problems that you've been having. Putting together all of the pieces of the problem helps us to make a treatment plan. This is a work in progress, so if I have anything wrong, please don't hesitate at all to let me know. My primary concern is helping you, so don't worry about speaking up if you want to clarify or add anything.

MICHAEL: Okay.

CLINICIAN: My sense is that what we are dealing with here is a great concern about making mistakes. This certainly fits with the social phobia—on a day-to-day basis, you are nervous about "messing up." Right?

MICHAEL: Yeah ... looking anxious, sounding anxious, saying the wrong thing, all that.

CLINICIAN: And what's so bad about these things [start of Socratic dialogue]?

MICHAEL: Well, if I look anxious, sound anxious, or say something stupid, people are going to think I am a fool and it will be pretty hard to ever change that impression.

CLINICIAN: And what would that mean for you?

MICHAEL: If I make a bad first impression, people won't want to spend time with me or come to my church services or work with me on class projects.

CLINICIAN: That sounds pretty rough.

MICHAEL: Yeah ... before I know it, I'll have no one. I'll be back in my pathology lab, just me and my tissue samples.

CLINICIAN: So, making mistakes has pretty dire consequences for you.

Kind of goes from perhaps making a bad impression to being sad and alone forever and ever more.

MICHAEL: Yeah. When I am sitting here, it sounds a little silly, but when I am in a social situation, the likelihood of messing up and suffering these consequences seems pretty realistic.

CLINICIAN: Yes . . . this is the social anxiety piece. But, am I correct in thinking it also fits in with the other things on the problem list?

MICHAEL: What do you mean?

CLINICIAN: Well, it seems to me that you are concerned with making mistakes in day-to-day life, but also with making mistakes about big "life decisions." If you enter the priesthood, will you regret disappointing your family or not having your own family? If you leave the priesthood and return to medicine, will you be regretful of that and worry about how you appear in God's eyes or in the eyes of your fellow seminarians? These would be big questions for anyone, but it seems that they get wrapped up a bit in the social anxiety. Right now, social anxiety clouds all of these decisions and, furthermore, might make you more concerned than other people about how others will react to your decisions.

MICHAEL: Wow. That's really right on the mark. All these random little problems do seem related.

CLINICIAN: Yes, the unifying theme seems to be a concern with making mistakes. Does this match your way of thinking about your situation?

MICHAEL: Well, I hadn't thought of it in this way, but now that you say it, I can really see it. But, what I don't see is what we *do* about it. I don't know if it is better to have a bunch of little unrelated problems or one colossal problem.

CLINICIAN: I can see your point. But I have some thoughts on what to do about it. Can I share them and see that you think?

MICHAEL: Sure.

Treatment Recommendations

CLINICIAN: Well, you came in asking for help with your social anxiety, so I think this is where we should start. Furthermore, it seems to me that making all of these life decisions could be complicated by social anxiety. For example, if you decided to leave the priesthood without first dealing with the social anxiety, you might always wonder if you left because of social anxiety or because it truly was not the "right" decision for you.

MICHAEL: I agree. Right now, any time I have the thought "Gee, this isn't for me," it's usually when I have something coming up that stirs up the anxiety.

CLINICIAN: Oh, that's interesting. That makes me even more confident that we need to work on the social anxiety first.

Informing the Client about the Specifics of Treatment to Obtain Consent

CLINICIAN: We are going to work on the social anxiety with a formal treatment protocol, designed specifically for clients with social phobia. The treatment typically runs for about 16 sessions, but we can be flexible. If some of the other problems are getting in the way of our progress with the program, we can deviate and deal with them. Similarly, if your social anxiety improves before the end of 16 sessions, we will "shift gears" and decide what to work on next.

MICHAEL: That sounds really good. I really like the plan.

CLINICIAN: Do you have any questions or thoughts about it?

MICHAEL: Well, you mentioned that we would treat the social phobia with a formal protocol. What does that involve?

CLINICIAN: We'll start with some psychoeducation. By this, I mean that you will learn some things about social phobia—how common it is, where it might come from, why it sticks around when you don't want to have it, and how we can treat it. Then we'll spend some time identifying the thoughts that cause your social anxiety and teach you some tools to challenge these thoughts. At that point, we get to the crux of the treatment—exposures. We will make a list of all of the situations that cause you difficulties and rate each according to how anxious it makes you feel. Then, in a systematic way, we will confront these situations.

MICHAEL: What do you mean, "Confront these situations"?

CLINICIAN: Yeah, sounds a little scary. Let me explain. A core technique of CBT is exposure to feared situations. By confronting situations that you have been avoiding, you will come to see that your anxiety will decrease with repeated exposures. Also, you will see that your feared consequences are pretty unlikely to occur, and if they were to occur, the consequences would not be as dire as you might expect.

MICHAEL: Can you give me an example?

CLINICIAN: We might have you give a sermon without preparing first.

MICHAEL: At all?!

CLINICIAN: We might try it in different ways. Maybe at first you could try it out with less preparation, and later on you could try it totally "off the cuff."

MICHAEL: That's impossible.

CLINICIAN: Might seem that way now. But that's why we do exposures gradually. We start with situations that cause moderate anxiety and we work up to those that cause a great deal of anxiety. By the time clients get to their most feared situations, they sometimes don't seem so scary anymore.

MICHAEL: So, you're telling me that if I did "off the cuff" sermons enough times, I'd get less and less anxious?

CLINICIAN: Probably. Any thoughts on why this could happen?

MICHAEL: I guess I'd learn that I wouldn't totally mess up.

CLINICIAN: Right. Here's another thing to think about, though. Even people who do a lot of public speaking might make a mistake from time to time. What would be the benefit of that happening to you?

MICHAEL: The benefit?

CLINICIAN: Yes, why might it actually be considered ideal for you to make a mistake?

MICHAEL: To show me that it's not that bad?

CLINICIAN: Right. Would you be kicked out the seminary for making a mistake? Would the parishioners heckle you?

MICHAEL: No. I see your point. You're trying to say that I wouldn't be rejected. But you wouldn't make me go out of my way to make a mistake, would you?

CLINICIAN: I don't "make" people do anything. But that is something I would suggest. Maybe you could intentionally pause for a moment or two, or say something wrong on purpose, or something like that. What do you think?

MICHAEL: I think that's crazy.

CLINICIAN: Okay. For a lot of clients, intentionally making a mistake has turned out to be a powerful learning experience. They really get to see that the consequences of making mistakes aren't that bad—and sometimes people don't even notice that they made a mistake at all. But let's just take the treatment step by step and see where we get to.

MICHAEL: I'll think it through, but I can't promise anything.

CLINICIAN: Fair enough.

MICHAEL: So, I am getting an idea of what we do with the social phobia. How do we deal with the other problems?

CLINICIAN: Well, a nice thing about CBT is that it provides a framework for dealing with all sorts of problems. During the social phobia program, you will learn how to identify negative thoughts and how to use specific tools to challenge these thoughts. These techniques will be really helpful when we start to work on some of the other problems as well. We can also pick and choose from other techniques that are encompassed by CBT. When we do work on your related problems, I think it will feel like quite a smooth transition from the social phobia treatment, since we will be approaching all of these issues from the same general perspective.

MICHAEL: That sounds really good.

Other Treatment Options

CLINICIAN: There are of course other options, too. You could consider taking medication to help the social anxiety. Is this something that you've considered?

MICHAEL: Yes, I've considered it. But, my preference would be to steer clear of medications for now. I don't have anything against them, but I like the idea of learning some new skills. If that doesn't work, then maybe we could talk some more about medications.

CLINICIAN: That is fine with me. Let me know along the way if you want to revisit the issue.

At this point, Michael was asked if he had any other questions or concerns. He did not, and at the end of the feedback session his clinician arranged for him to come back the next week for his first session of treatment.

ADDRESSING COMMONLY ASKED QUESTIONS ABOUT CBT

Before concluding this chapter and moving on to the process of CBT, let's review some commonly asked questions that come up when clients are considering options for treatment. Some clients will hear your brief overview of CBT, see it as worth trying, and "sign on." Others will follow your overview with questions and concerns. It is important to spend the time answering them and providing clients with the information that they need to make an informed decision about treatment.

"Does CBT Work?"

Many clients (understandably) will ask if CBT "works." Although some clients will seek out CBT because they have learned about its efficacy from other sources, others will be hearing about it for the first time during their initial contact with mental health professionals. Since CBT sounds so different from the notion of psychotherapy held by most lay people, they might be doubtful about its validity or efficacy. Having confidence in the treatment approach can have an impact on therapy outcome, so it is very important to try to instill some of the confidence that we feel about CBT in our clients.

This can be difficult for beginning clinicians, who sometimes feel pressure to "sell" CBT to prospective clients. They might worry that if they "pitch" the treatment and clients decide not to pursue it, they will be negatively evaluated by their supervisors. It is important, then, to strike a balance between providing clients with information that will help them to make an appropriate decision about treatment, while not pushing them into a treatment program that they do not want to enter.

There are two ways that this "hard sell" can be avoided. First, stick to the facts. Tell clients that CBT is an empirically supported approach to treatment. Give them specific information about the effectiveness of CBT for their particular difficulties. Let clients know that CBT is not a new approach to treatment, but rather has been used to treat psychological disorders for over four decades. If true, it can also be beneficial to mention that you have treated other clients (being mindful of confidentiality, of course) with similar problems who did well with CBT.

Second, come back to the stance of collaborative empiricism. It is fine to share with clients your confidence in CBT, but to also appreciate their doubts. After all, you have seen CBT work effectively, and they have not. Clients can be encouraged to try CBT and see how it works. While their hypothesis might be that CBT will not work for them, they can be encouraged to reevaluate how things are going at a certain point in time (e.g., at the midpoint in an agreed-upon course of therapy) and see whether or not their hypothesis has garnered support. Regardless, it is critical that clients be open to the possibility that CBT *might* work for them; it would be unreasonable to expect clients to have complete confidence in the approach until they have given it a try.

A good way to have this discussion with clients is to ask if they remember what it was like to learn something new that they now do with little effort. Most people can remember learning to spell their name or learning to tie their shoes. Other clients might recall what it was like to learn a new language or sport or how to play a musical instrument. Consider a client who presented with a specific phobia of driving:

CLIENT: I can't imagine ever getting to the point where I feel fine about driving. I've been trying hard to get past it, but it's just impossible.

CLINICIAN: Have you ever tried to learn something new that seemed impossible when you first got started?

CLIENT: Hmmmm. I guess learning French. My husband is from France and he's fluent in English, but most of his relatives just speak French. So, when we got engaged, I decided I should learn French since we were going to visit there after our wedding. I wanted to be able to speak to his family.

CLINICIAN: How did you learn to speak French?

CLIENT: Well, I first got a tape. I'd listen on my headphones when I was walking from place to place and I did okay with learning things like introducing myself or asking for directions or ordering food in a restaurant. But then I'd get home and hear my husband chatting away on the phone with his relatives and have no idea what they were talking about. It was so discouraging!

CLINICIAN: So, what did you do?

CLIENT: Well, then I enrolled in a class at the university. I had a choice of a few different places, but I chose a class where the teacher said he'd be speaking virtually no English at all! He said it was the best way to learn.

CLINICIAN: And, how did it go?

CLIENT: At first, terribly! I was so lost. I had no idea what was going on for the first 2 weeks. But, then I started to catch on. I really started practicing at home too with my husband. And, I'd say that within 6 months, I was in good shape. I'm pretty fluent now—I get confused once in a while or say the wrong thing, but nothing too terrible.

CLINICIAN: When you first bought that tape, would you have expected you'd get this far?

CLIENT: No way! It just felt impossible. But I plugged away and worked really hard and it paid off.

CLINICIAN: Do you see any connection between your experiences with French and getting over your driving fears?

CLIENT: Well, it is funny. I bought a self-help book, but it hasn't helped me. I still can't get in the car. I guess it's the same as my tape. It wasn't till I took a class that I started to really learn to speak French.

CLINICIAN: So?

CLIENT: So, I guess if you and I work on this together, it might really be of help. I guess it's not fair to judge until I give it a try.

CLINICIAN: Is there anything else about your experiences with learning French that might help you here?

CLIENT: Well, I guess I have to remember that it won't be easy right away. I have to work at it and kind of have reasonable expectations.

CLINICIAN: I think that is an excellent way to look at it.

"Will We Have Enough Time to Work on My Problems?"

Clients can have different reactions to learning that CBT is time-limited. Many clients view this positively—it is comforting to know that their problems will not take years to resolve. Furthermore, the time-limited nature of CBT can be very motivating for clients. If a therapy assignment seems overwhelming, but clients know that they only have a few months to work on their difficulties, they might be more willing to push themselves to try difficult things.

Some clients, however, worry that the duration of therapy will not be sufficient for them to make the improvements they would like to make. It is easy to understand these concerns, particularly with clients who have been having difficulties for many years. It is hard to imagine working through a problem in a couple of months that has been around for 30 years. It can be helpful here to return to what we know from research and from our experiences with other clients. CBT has been shown to be effective when carried out in a time-limited fashion, even with clients who present with severe and long-lasting symptoms. This information should be presented to clients, but it is not necessary to try to convince them that time-limited treatment will work for them, too. Rather, return to the empirical stance of CBT and encourage them to be scientists—"Why don't we get started with this plan and see how things go?" Another helpful message to deliver to clients is that CBT involves ongoing consideration and revision of the case conceptualization. The plan for treatment is not written in stone and is frequently evaluated and revised as the therapy progresses.

"Why Didn't CBT Work for Me in the Past?"

Sometimes clients have previously undergone CBT and experienced little or no improvement. In this situation, you should spend some time ascertaining the exact nature of the previous treatment. Often, you can quite clearly identify a reason for the treatment failure.

Sometimes clients think they have received CBT, but when they begin to describe what their treatment entailed, it is clear that they received something else altogether. Some clients might have received only certain components of CBT (e.g., only cognitive work without the behavioral component). They might not have had an adequate trial of CBT (e.g., they stayed in therapy for only four sessions when CBT for many disorders takes longer than that to start working). Some clients might have received very good CBT for an adequate period of time, but other variables might have influenced its efficacy. CBT is a treatment that requires a commitment of time and effort on the part of a client, and some clients will clearly tell you that the last time they tried CBT, they were not ready to change or did not have the time to commit to getting well. Securing information of this sort from the client is very important. Using a cognitive-behavioral approach, misconceptions can quite quickly be remedied, placing clients in a better mindset for beginning CBT again.

On a related note, some clients say that they have tried to implement CBT techniques on their own—with little success. Either with a self-help book, or through intuition, clients might have tried to challenge their thoughts, expose themselves to something they are afraid of, or replace an unhealthy behavior with one that is more adaptive. They might wonder why formal CBT will work, if their own efforts had not. A good way to respond to this concern is to first commend clients for their efforts. Their experiences can then be normalized—most clients have tried to improve their lot in life on their own prior to coming for treatment. However, if it were so easy to change the way that one thinks and behaves, people would not have any problems!

One of the strengths of therapy is that the clinicians can help clients to understand the contingencies that maintain their problematic thoughts and behaviors and can then teach them specific strategies for making desired changes. A good example to consider is dieting—many people try to lose weight on their own and fail. They might decide to eat less and exercise more, but in reality, cannot accomplish these goals. The advantage of therapy is that it helps clients to articulate *specific* changes that must be made to meet these elusive goals. Treatment might start with helping the client to identify triggers for overeating and roadblocks that get in the way of exercising—in other words, identifying the factors that maintain the weight problem in the first place. Then the therapist can help the client develop a specific plan for eating less and exercising more. If a trigger for overeating is being bored and alone in the evenings, the therapist might help the client develop a number of ways to alleviate boredom (e.g., get some good books to read; work on a home improvement project) and reduce loneliness (e.g., join an organization; do some volunteer work; get together with friends to see a movie). The therapist can also help the client examine his or her eating habits and identify positive changes that can be made. If the client eats a healthy dinner at 5 P.M. and then binges on junk food at 11 P.M., the therapist might suggest having dinner a little later in the evening and then also planning to have a healthy snack later on. Similarly, the therapist might help the client develop an exercise plan that takes into account the roadblocks that previously interfered. If the client does not like exercising in a gym, he or she can be encouraged to find a nice walking route in the neighborhood. A client who finds it hard to get motivated to exercise alone could be encouraged to find an "exercise buddy," which could also reduce his or her feelings of boredom and loneliness. As these potential solutions are generated and applied, the therapist can help the client evaluate the results and consider other alternative solutions if the initial plan did not work. In other words, rather than giving up after one night of overeating or a missed day of exercise, therapy provides the structure for persevering with solving a problem. Clients generally appreciate being commended for trying to solve their problems on their own, and are usually quite able to see how a structured cognitive-behavioral approach, with a supportive clinician, might lead to better results.

"Should I Take Medication?"

Particularly since pharmaceutical companies have started to advertise on television and in popular magazines, many clients come to see clinicians with numerous questions about medication. It is not unusual for clients to come in having diagnosed themselves and having selected a medication that they think might be of help to them. Despite the fact that most clinicians cannot prescribe medication, it is extremely important to be knowledgeable about them and to be able to answer the questions that clients ask.

Clients ask some pretty standard questions on this topic, mostly along the theme of the comparable efficacy of therapy, medication, or combined treatments. Although this is perhaps an overgeneralization, many treatment outcome studies across disorders suggest that therapy and medication are about equally effective, but that medication tends to work a bit faster and therapy tends to have better long-term efficacy. The research on combined treatments is a bit more complicated, with some studies showing that combined treatments are more effective than either treatment approach alone and some showing no advantage of combined treatment.

As a clinician, a good way for you to manage this kind of question is to take the client's lifestyle into account. Explain the pros and cons of each approach to clients and reassess their views once they have the appropriate information. The advantage of both approaches is that they are effective. Now, more than ever, we have effective therapeutic approaches and medications to treat some of the most common psychological disorders.

Like therapy, medication also has some drawbacks. All medications have side effects, and clients must be made aware of these. Medication can be very expensive, particularly for clients without health insurance. As with therapy, the use of medication also requires strict adherence to a treatment regimen. In contrast to therapy, medication use may not be time-limited, but clients should know that taking medication alone might be associated with poorer long-term efficacy than receiving therapy alone. Clinicians and clients should work together to come up with the best treatment approach given the clients' difficulties and life-style related factors. In Chapter 7, we discuss in much greater detail issues related to doing CBT and taking medication concurrently.

WRITING THE REPORT

Once you have worked through the process of case conceptualization and have devised an initial treatment plan, you will be ready to write your assessment report. There are many different ways to write an assessment report, and most agencies will have templates for you to follow of the way that they like reports to be written. In general, certain information should be included in reports regardless of the specific format (see Groth-Marnat, 1997).

Some General Rules for Report Writing

One of the most important rules of report writing is to be succinct. You do not have to put *everything* into the report that you learned during the assessment. Carefully select the information that is going to best capture the client, keeping in mind that other professionals are very busy and want to get a clear picture of the client as quickly as possible. Furthermore, when clients read their own reports, they can often feel overwhelmed with too much information. Keeping it simple and providing straightforward recommendations is strongly encouraged.

It is also important to be mindful of your audience. The report's audience should help you to determine what to put into it. This issue is most salient when reports are being sent to other people in clients' lives. For example, if an employer requests an assessment to see if an employee is able to work, the report should focus on factors relevant to this assessment question. Highly personal information about relationships, sexual orientation, family history, and other issues like these typically do not have a place in such reports and should be excluded even if brought up during the assessment.

Be mindful that clients have a right to see their own reports. This does not mean you cannot be honest about difficult issues—rather, you should word your comments to be helpful, but not harmful, to clients. For example, if a client is very chatty during an assessment, it would not be helpful to write, "The client would not stop talking through the entire interview." Rather, you might write, "The client seemed to have some difficulty answering questions succinctly during the interview." You should also be mindful of the language that you use, avoiding jargon. This is also important when communicating with other professionals who might not be knowledgeable about mental health or the cognitive-behavioral approach to treatment. If clients do want to see their reports, it is best for clinicians to review the report with them and be available to address any questions or concerns that may arise.

Let's now look briefly at each main section that should be included in the standard report. In Figure 5.1, we have included a sample report based on the case of Michael to demonstrate these key features.

General Information

The report should begin with the client's name, age/date of birth, and sex. It should also include the date of the assessment, the date the report was written, and the name of the evaluator. Finally, information should be provided about the referral source.

Referral Question

According to Groth-Marnat (1997), "The 'referral question' section provides a brief description of the client and a statement of the general reason for conducting the evaluation" (p. 632). This should be a brief section, basically orienting the reader to the content of the remainder of the report. A full description of the client can be put in the "Background Information" section. In this section, the purpose of the evaluation should be indicated. In Michael's case, he had contacted the clinic on his own (without a referral from another professional), desiring help with his social anxiety.

Evaluation Procedures

In this section, the evaluation instruments that were used should be listed and briefly described. Acronyms should not be used until the full

FIGURE 5.1. Sample report for Michael.

Name: Michael J.
Date of birth: June 8, 1963
Age: 40
Sex: Male
Date of assessment: April 6, 2004
Date of report: April 10, 2004
Clinician: Dr. T.
Referral source: Self-referred

Referral Question: Michael is a 40-year-old, white, single male who presented with complaints of social anxiety, particularly around public speaking.

Evaluation Procedures: Michael was administered the *Structured Clinical Interview for DSM-IV (SCID-IV)*. The SCID-IV assesses for the presence of anxiety disorders, mood disorders, substance use disorders, somatoform disorders, eating disorders, and also includes a screen for psychotic symptoms.

Michael was sent a battery of questionnaires completed by all clients who present at our clinic. The battery includes a number of measures assessing anxiety and mood difficulties. Focus here will be placed on measures of social anxiety and depression:

Beck Depression Inventory (BDI-II): The BDI is the most commonly-used self-report measure of depressive affect. The 21-item scale assesses symptoms of depression that have been present in the past week including difficulties with sleep, irritability and suicidal ideation.

Social Phobia Scale (SPS): The SPS is a 20-item self-report measure that assesses fear of being scrutinized during routine activities like eating or writing in front of others.

Social Interaction Anxiety Scale (SIAS): The SIAS is a 20-item self-report measure that assesses cognitive, affective, and behavioral reactions to social interactions.

Michael came to the evaluation with his self-report measures completed. The assessment interview took 2 hours to complete.

Behavioral Observations: Michael arrived for his appointment slightly early. He was neatly groomed and looked slightly younger than his 40 years. He seemed quite anxious at the beginning of the interview, but as it progressed, he became more comfortable. Michael is a very intelligent, articulate man and was able to answer all of the questions posed to him in a clear, concise manner. Although slightly reluctant to discuss very personal matters (e.g., decisions about having a family), he was for the most part very open about sharing his concerns and experiences. The assessor had no concerns about the reliability of the information that Michael provided.

Background Information: Michael was born in New England. He grew up in a home with both of his parents and his younger sister, Mary. Both of his parents are still living and in reasonably good health. Mary is married, has four children, and lives near their parents. For the most part, the family gets along quite well, and Michael visits them a number of times each year for holidays and other family events. There is no history of mental health problems in the family.

(*continued on next page*)

FIGURE 5.1. (*continued*)

Michael reports having had a good childhood. He had some friends (fewer than other children had, according to him) and excelled at school. He was quite involved in church, but being serious about his studies, he engaged in few other extracurricular activities. After graduating from college with a degree in chemistry, Michael attended medical school and became a pathologist. He worked for the past number of years at the same medical center, eventually being appointed head of the Pathology Department. During his adult years, Michael had done some dating, but he had never had a serious relationship. He explained that he had little time for dating, due to the demands of his job. Upon questioning, he conceded that social anxiety had also prevented him from dating, particularly as he got older and was meeting fewer people. When he was not working, he dedicated much of his free time to the church, attending services and volunteering with disadvantaged children in his community.

Approximately 3 years ago, Michael attended a church retreat at which he felt he was called to the priesthood. He considered this path seriously, and 4 months ago took a leave of absence from his job and started his novitiate year, in which he would study and consider the priesthood. He is currently living at the seminary. At the time that he presented for treatment, Michael explained that his social anxiety—which had always been a problem—had started to cause him a great deal more distress than it had in the past number of years. In his new role he has to do a lot of public speaking, in church services as well as in the classroom. He is also meeting many more new people than he has in recent years, and these more casual interactions are also distressing for Michael.

Michael described having been socially anxious for as long as he can remember. He recalls always having been shy with peers, particularly with girls, as he got older. He also experienced a great deal of anxiety in school when he had to do public speaking, fearing that the other students would tease him for blushing. Michael experienced a lot of distress in medical school as well when he was put on the spot and asked questions in front of other medical students, superiors, and patients. He explained that he chose pathology as a specialty because it involved very little interaction with others. For the past number of years, he worked at the same hospital, dated very little, and did minimal socializing outside of church (where he felt quite comfortable), allowing him to keep his social anxiety at bay. In his current role, he is experiencing significant social anxiety every day and spending a great deal of time (over) preparing for class presentations, sermons, and so forth in order to decrease the likelihood that he will make mistakes. He avoids more casual social interactions when possible; when he does socialize, he pays careful attention to how he is coming across. This includes monitoring what he is saying, reviewing what he has just said to see if anything sounded "dumb," and considering how hot his face feels to see if he is blushing. These behaviors make it very difficult for Michael to attend to conversations.

Other than his difficulties with social anxiety, Michael reported good mental and physical health.

Assessment Results: On the SCID, criteria were met only for social phobia, generalized subtype. Criteria were not met for any other current or lifetime diagnoses. Michael's self-report measures were in line with these findings. His BDI score was low, suggesting that depression is not a problem for him right now. He scored slightly above the mean for clinical samples on both the SIAS and SPS. On other measures of anxiety-related concerns (worry, panic, obsessions and compulsions), Michael scored within the normal range.

(*continued on next page*)

FIGURE 5.1. (*continued*)

Impressions: Michael is currently experiencing moderately severe social phobia, as well as some conflicts about the choices he is facing in his personal and professional life. Despite these challenges, Michael is functioning quite well right now. Overtly, he is avoiding relatively little, but he experiences a great deal of distress in social situations. To deal with this distress, and to prevent negative outcomes (e.g., social rejection), Michael engages in numerous subtle avoidance strategies while in social situations (e.g., carefully considering what to say) and in anticipation of them (e.g., overpreparing).

Recommendations: Cognitive-behavioral therapy (CBT) for social phobia will likely be a good starting point for Michael. It seems important to help him learn to manage his anxiety better in social situations so that he can focus on making decisions based on what he wants from life, rather than on the influence of his social anxiety. Once Michael feels better able to cope with social situations, he can begin to explore the choices that are facing him in both his personal and professional life. Michael seems to be an excellent candidate for CBT. He has good insight into his difficulties, he is bright, and he is most certainly motivated to work on his social anxiety and to explore the challenges that are currently facing him.

Options for medication were discussed with Michael. At the present time, Michael is not interested in trying pharmacological treatment for social phobia. It was our impression that medication is not necessary at this time for Michael.

---

name of the instrument is introduced. Once an acronym is defined (e.g., Beck Depression Inventory; BDI), it can be used in the remainder of the report. It can be helpful in this section to indicate how long the assessment took to complete. Such information can be important for case conceptualization and treatment planning.

Behavioral Observations

Focus should be placed in this section on the client's appearance, observations of behavior before, during and after the evaluation, and the nature of the interactions between the client and clinician. Connections should also be drawn between these observations and the validity of the evaluation. If a client is very argumentative and oppositional during the evaluation and provides information that seems incongruent with his or her behavior, this should be noted.

Background Information

This section of the report should include information on family background, personal history, medical history, history of the problem, and current life situation (see Groth-Marnat, 1997). It is very important that this section be written succinctly. Other professionals are just as busy as you are, and the information that they need to help the client should be delivered in a concise and organized fashion. Instead of elucidating every aspect of the client's life, focus on information that is relevant to the client's current difficulties. Groth-Marnat (1997) has recommended that report writers be clear about the sources of their information. For example, a report might read, "According to the client . . . " or "Discussion with the client's mother revealed that. . . . "

Assessment Results

In this section, findings from each assessment tool listed in the "Evaluation Procedures" section are reported. It is beyond the scope of this book to provide an in-depth discussion of how to describe test results (e.g., from intelligence tests). When discussing Michael's case, we noted the diagnosis for which he met criteria and reported the results of his self-report measures in the context of normative data. One general rule of thumb when reporting assessment results is to avoid reporting raw scores whenever possible. Writing that Michael scored 4 on the BDI, 46 on the Social Phobia Scale (SPS) and 28 on the Social Interaction Anxiety Scale (SIAS) is meaningless to everyone except the relatively small number of people who are familiar with these measures. In order to get around this problem, verbal interpretations are preferred ("His BDI score indicated minimal depression"). Alternatively, scores can be compared to normative data. On the SPS and SIAS, Michael scored slightly above the mean reported by clinical samples of persons with social phobia in the published literature, but his scores on other measures that he completed were similar to those reported by nonclinical samples. Such statements are much more meaningful than raw scores to individuals reading reports (including clients themselves).

Impression and Interpretations

This section should summarize what was learned from the assessment process. It should integrate test data, behavioral observations, relevant history, and any other data, such as information from other professionals or family members (Groth-Marnat, 1997). We have purposefully written a very brief impression and interpretation section, since this section will vary greatly depending on the setting in which you work. In some settings, this section might include a case formulation as described by Persons. In others, it might be less interpretive (as we have done here). Here, we have addressed Michael's general level of psychopathology, focusing specifically on both the distress that he is experiencing and the degree to which his social anxiety is leading to functional impairment.

Recommendations

Again, this section will read very differently depending on your orientation and the setting in which you work. Here, we have recommended CBT, have discussed how treatment for Michael's problems might be sequenced, and have made a statement on how we expect that he will do in CBT. We also noted that medication options were discussed with Michael, but that he was not eager to try medication at this time. Table 5.2 summarizes what should be included in the assessment report.

TABLE 5.2. Information to Include in an Assessment Report

1. General information
   • Client's name, date of birth/age, sex
   • Date of assessment, date the report was written, name of evaluator, referral source

2. Referral question
   • Brief description of the client
   • Reason for conducting the evaluation

3. Evaluation procedures
   • Names and brief descriptions of evaluation instruments to be used
   • Length of the assessment

4. Behavioral observations
   • Appearance
   • General behavioral observations
   • Nature of the interaction between the client and clinician

5. Background information
   • Family background
   • Personal history
   • Medical history
   • History of the problem
   • Current life situation

6. Assessment results
   • List findings from each assessment tool.

7. Impression and interpretations
   • Summarize what was learned during the assessment.

8. Recommendations
   • Indicate whether or not treatment is recommended.
   • If treatment is recommended, note what kind(s) of treatment are recommended and why.
   • If there are multiple problems, note which one to focus on first.

9. Comment on prognosis

Chapter 6

■ ■ ■

STARTING THE COGNITIVE-BEHAVIORAL TREATMENT PROCESS

In some settings, you will begin therapy with a client who has already been assessed by someone else. When this occurs, it is important to acquaint yourself with the case before the first session by carefully reviewing the chart and discussing the case with the clinician who did the assessment. Try to get a sense of what the client's life is like and try to gain a clear picture of the difficulties for which he or she is seeking help. As you get acquainted with the case, it can be helpful to jot down some questions that you would like to ask the client during the initial session based on your reading and discussion with the clinician who did the assessment.

If you assessed the client whom you will treat, it is still important to review the chart before the first session, in order to become reacquainted with the details of the client's life and the kinds of difficulties he or she is having. For clinicians who see many clients at any given time, or when some time has elapsed between assessment and first session of treatment, these details can become hazy. It would be quite offensive to clients if you had forgotten major details about their lives after you had spent many hours with them during the assessment process. The establishment of rapport is much better served if you can start the session with a few personal questions such as "How are your children doing?" or "How did that presentation at work that you were telling me about when you were in last time end up going?"

THE IMPORTANCE OF SETTING AN AGENDA

As treatment planning is to the overall course of therapy, agenda setting is to each individual session of therapy. Agenda setting occurs both behind the scenes and in the room with clients. A rough agenda should be set by the clinician before going into each session with the client. The basic framework for a generic session of CBT is outlined in Table 6.1. The agenda should cue the clinician to check in about the week, review homework, and assign homework for the following week. Between reviewing completed homework and assigning new homework, the meat of the session occurs.

As we discussed in the last chapter, clinicians embark on a course of treatment having a general sense of what will happen from session to session (i.e., what will happen in "the meat" of each session). This decision is often derived from a therapy manual. For example, Michael's initial Treatment Plan, which was outlined in Table 4.2, lists the particular main content scheduled in each session, starting off with psychoeducational information. This general framework, though, does not tell the clinician what the exact content of each session will be (e.g., what exposures to do, what kinds of dysfunctional thoughts to work on, etc.). These decisions are based on our experiences from session to session. Our understanding of cases is fluid, changing from session to session as we get to know our clients better. This growing understanding (and our constantly evolving case conceptualization) should inform the treatment plan from week to week.

While clinicians must give some thought to the content of the session before it begins (and discuss the plan with a supervisor, where applicable), it is essential that clients be involved in planning sessions as well. Each session should begin with the clinician checking in with the client and asking "What should we put on our agenda for today?" Clinicians can then help clients to develop an agenda that can be put to good use.

TABLE 6.1. A Basic Treatment Session Agenda

1. Check in with the client about week.
2. Collaboratively set the session agenda.
3. Review homework.
4. Conduct main session content based on treatment plan.
5. Assign new homework (usually based on main session content).
6. Summarize session with the client (ask the client what he or she learned).
7. Check in with the client (any questions, concerns, other issues to discuss?).

Clients sometimes list so many issues that if all were put on the agenda, none could be covered adequately. Clinicians can help their clients to select the few most important issues to put on the agenda for that day and then help them to figure out what to do with the remaining issues. Some "leftover" issues could be developed into homework assignments; others could be tabled for the following week.

Between sessions, "life happens." Clients often come in to sessions wanting to discuss an issue that does not follow from what happened in the previous session or from what was planned for the current one. It is the clinician's job to figure out how flexible to be about the agenda. In some cases, it would be clinically irresponsible not to devote time to the new issue. Clients suffer losses, have fights with significant others, and can also have nice things happen like pregnancies or promotions at work. Shifting away from the agreed-upon plan for part of a session or an entire session is fine, and, in fact, it is quite uncommon to complete a whole course of therapy and never have this occur.

As we discuss in greater detail in Chapter 9, some clients come in to virtually every session wanting to discuss some "crisis" that happened during the week. This is problematic if it diverts attention from other, more important issues. In fact, such behavior may be conceptualized as a way to avoid working on difficult material. Obviously, we want to keep clients on track and help them to work on the issues for which they sought treatment, yet we also want to balance this with maintaining rapport. If clients come in each week with issues to discuss that we do not allow them to add to the agenda, they might feel misunderstood and frustrated with the rigidity of treatment. An ideal solution to this problem is to spend a limited amount of time on the new issue at the beginning of the session, deciding if it needs to be attended to immediately or if it should be tabled for the following session.

THE FIRST TREATMENT SESSION

Introductions, Reviews, and Check-Ins

The first session of most CBT protocols consists of covering psychoeducational material. Although we want to make sure to have sufficient time to cover this area, it is also terribly important during all therapy sessions (particularly early ones) to be mindful of the therapeutic relationship. For the first treatment session, if you have not met the client, a general rule is to introduce yourself and allow the client to introduce him- or herself, too. Ask clients how they are doing that day or since the last time you have met. Let them know that you are looking forward to working with them.

At the beginning of the first session, the clinician and the client should briefly review the presenting problems, and clients should be asked if anything has changed since their assessment appointment. For example, clients with depression can be asked how their mood has been and clients with substance use problems can be asked about their pattern of use since they last saw you. Some clients might also want to discuss how they felt about the assessment and how they feel about starting treatment. For some clients, going through an assessment, receiving feedback, and being given recommendations for treatment can be extremely beneficial. These clients might come in for their first postassessment session saying that they feel very hopeful about making positive changes in their lives. For other clients, the assessment process can be quite dispiriting. It can be extremely difficult and painful for some clients to speak about their difficulties. By getting it all "out on the table," so to speak, some clients might feel as if their difficulties are too serious and too overwhelming to be "fixed." These comments should not be ignored, since clients' beliefs about their ability to change can have a significant impact on treatment outcome. Some time should be spent correcting the client's misconceptions about therapy (e.g., "I think my problems are too severe for CBT") and providing them with some hope about their prognosis.

Providing an Overview of the Treatment

At this point, clients should be given an idea of what the treatment program will entail. This serves to set the agenda not only for the session but for the treatment program as a whole. They might have already heard this treatment description—perhaps during their initial phone call to the clinic, or in the feedback session, or perhaps when speaking to their clinician about setting up an initial session. It is a good idea, though, to review it briefly, as it affords clients the opportunity to ask questions about the program. Let's return to the case of Michael to illustrate how to give such an overview:

CLINICIAN: So Michael, now that we've spent some time catching up on how things have been going for you these last few weeks, let's talk about the treatment program that we are going to be working on together. We spoke about it a little bit at our feedback session, but let's get into more detail today so that you have a sense of how the therapy will progress.

MICHAEL: Okay.

CLINICIAN: Starting today, we will be spending some time learning more about social anxiety—how common it is, what causes it, and how we go about treating it. We'll get started with this material today and will spend some of the next session finishing it.

After we finish this educational material, we will work together to build a "fear and avoidance hierarchy." This is a list of the social situations that are difficult for you, that are arranged in order from least to most anxiety-provoking. This hierarchy will guide the work that we do together. We will start by working on situations that are moderately difficult for you, and as you gain confidence and learn new ways to think about social situations, we will gradually move up the hierarchy to the more anxiety-provoking items.

MICHAEL: How soon will that come? I mean, how soon are you going to make me do all of these things?

CLINICIAN: Good question. Let me address one thing you said before I answer it, though. You just asked me how soon I am going to "make" you do all of these frightening things. I actually won't be "making" you do anything. This is a collaborative endeavor. While I will certainly make suggestions about how the therapy should proceed, you will be an active participant. I will certainly encourage you to do tough things, but I won't make you do anything.

MICHAEL: That's a relief.

CLINICIAN: What I will do is try to demonstrate to you why I think doing the "hard" things is important when we get to them. Returning to your question, we will be doing our first exposure in Session 5. After we develop the hierarchy, but before we get to actually doing exposures, we will spend a few sessions exploring your thoughts about social situations. This is the cognitive part of CBT that we talked about before.

MICHAEL: Oh right. So—identifying thoughts and then fixing ones up that aren't very helpful for me.

CLINICIAN: Yes, that's the idea. Our thoughts can be quite detrimental and we need to get good at identifying negative thoughts, exploring them to see if they are rational and helpful to us, and if they aren't, we need to work on reframing them to be more rational and helpful. So, we'll spend some sessions on that and then we will apply what we've learned to actually getting into social situations.

MICHAEL: Okay.

CLINICIAN: Now, by the time we start doing exposures, will anything be different that might make them seem less scary than they seem right now?

MICHAEL: Well, we would have done the cognitive work. So, presumably I might be thinking a bit differently than I think right now. That could be helpful.

CLINICIAN: Absolutely. Is there anything else that might make things a bit easier to handle that we would have done earlier in treatment?

MICHAEL: Well, I would have learned a bit more about social anxiety. Maybe this would make me feel less bad that I have the problem. Oh, and the hierarchy. It's going to be gradual, so we'll start with things that aren't that nerve-wracking for me.

CLINICIAN: Right. You've made two excellent points. So, let's talk a bit more about these exposures. We'll start out doing the first exposure together in one of our sessions. It will be something reasonably low on your hierarchy. Then, we'll discuss an exposure that you can do on your own for homework. The rest of our sessions will be structured in much the same way—reviewing how homework went, doing some exposures in our sessions, and then deciding on homework for the following week.

MICHAEL: How long does that last?

CLINICIAN: In total, the therapy runs between 16 and 20 sessions. There is certainly some flexibility there. Some people make progress quickly and end treatment earlier. Some people need a few extra sessions tacked on at the end. We'll see how it goes, but we do typically finish up treatment by Session 20. I should also mention that we do some special things at the end of treatment to help you maintain the gains you've made in treatment once you are done.

MICHAEL: Well, that all sounds good. A little scary, but it makes sense.

CLINICIAN: Any questions?

MICHAEL: Not for right now.

CLINICIAN: Please don't hesitate to ask. Some clients, particularly those with social anxiety, worry about asking questions for fear that the clinician will judge them negatively. It's also pretty common for clients to be anxious early in therapy, and their anxiety can make it harder to pay attention. It's totally fine to ask questions or ask me to repeat things that seemed unclear.

MICHAEL: Thanks. I appreciate that. I think I'm good for now. Sometimes I think of things after the fact, once I have time to mull things over. So, I guess I could scribble down questions that I have during the week and bring them in next time.

CLINICIAN: That would be great.

As a general rule, it is best to keep the overview of treatment brief and simple. Clients will get the clearest sense of how treatment works once they start to do it. Perhaps the most important part of providing this overview is inviting clients to ask questions and to voice concerns. There are two general tips to keep in mind with respect to clients' questions and concerns about treatment. First, whenever possible, use Socratic questioning to help clients respond to their own concerns. Obviously, some questions are best answered directly (e.g., how long therapy lasts, what the word hierarchy means, etc.). In other cases, Socratic questioning can be very useful, as demonstrated previously, when Michael voiced concern about doing exposures to feared social situations. Rather than trying to convince Michael that the exposures would not be scary or agreeing with him that they would be scary, his clinician posed a question to see if he could think more rationally about the idea (e.g., "Will anything be different then that might make social situations seem less scary than they seem right now?"). By taking this stance, clients begin very early on to start seeing the relationship between thoughts and behaviors and start to recognize the utility of challenging their beliefs.

The previously presented dialogue also demonstrated how important it is to address clients' reluctance to ask questions and/or voice concerns in therapy. Normalizing this fear (e.g., "A lot of clients feel nervous about asking questions") and letting clients know that they should feel comfortable asking questions has a very positive impact on the therapeutic relationship and, most likely, on treatment outcome as well.

Sharing Knowledge: The Psychoeducation Component of Treatment

Why Do Psychoeducation?

Most CBT programs start out by sharing with clients some educational material. Some beginning clinicians, and sometimes clients themselves, see psychoeducation as a "waste of time." They wonder why they are not just jumping into the meat of therapy. Despite this desire, there are many advantages to spending a session or two covering this material. First, it can be helpful in terms of establishing rapport. Psychoeducation can be viewed as a learning process shared by the client and the clinician. As clinicians educate clients about the nature of the problems they are having and how to best treat them, clients should be kept involved. Rather than lecturing, clinicians should continually ask clients how particular concepts apply to them. This allows for the clinician to also get "up to speed" on the problems that the client is experiencing and informs the ongoing case conceptualization. This process demonstrates to the client that he or she is a crucial part of the treatment team. When clients feel as if they are playing an integral role in their treatment, they are usually more motivated to work on their difficulties.

As clients share their experiences, there is also an opportunity for clinicians to normalize these experiences. For example, a clinician can tell clients about the prevalence rates of the kinds of problems they are having or can let clients know that he or she has treated many other individuals with similar problems. Clients are often amazed to hear that others share their experiences. Rapport is undoubtedly strengthened when clinicians seem familiar and comfortable with the problems being described to them.

On the other hand, we do not want clients to feel that we are minimizing their problems, or communicating that treatment is not necessary. Psychoeducation can also afford the opportunity to discuss with clients how their problems are interfering in their functioning. Again, this serves to strengthen rapport since it makes the client feel that the therapist understands his or her day-to-day struggles. By also initiating a discussion about how life might be better for clients after completing treatment, psychoeducation can serve a motivating function, particularly for clients who are "on the fence" about whether or not to engage in treatment.

One final strength of psychoeducation (and, again, a reason why it strengthens rapport) is that it is a relatively nonthreatening means of interacting. Rather than being asked immediately to eat a forbidden food or touch something perceived to be contaminated, clients are given an opportunity to acclimate to the therapy environment. This time allows for the client to gain confidence in the clinician and in the treatment program before the "real" work of therapy begins.

What Should Psychoeducation Consist of?

The specific content of psychoeducation sessions will vary, depending on the problems for which the client is seeking help. For example, Michael's psychoeducation session will focus on what science knows about social anxiety and social phobia. However, regardless of the specific disorder, there are some commonalities simply because psychoeducation serves a common function: to get clients "on board" with the CBT approach to understanding and treating their particular difficulties. To meet this goal, clients should be presented with the cognitive-behavioral model for understanding the disorder and/or problem for which they are seeking treatment. Most disorder-specific treatment manuals include a cognitive-behavioral model for understanding that particular disorder (a list of cognitive-behavioral treatment manuals for various disorders is included in Appendix A).

A good way to explain the model for a specific disorder is to draw a diagram as the client looks on. Using a whiteboard or a chalkboard can be helpful. For example, the cognitive-behavioral model of social anxiety has three components: the cognitive, the physiological, and the behavioral (this likely reminds you of the bottom portion of Figure 1.1, The Cognitive Model). These components can be described as the way clients think, feel in the body, and behave. As each component is added to the model, clients should be asked how it might apply to them. After the model has been introduced, a discussion can ensue about how specific treatment techniques (e.g., cognitive restructuring, exposure, behavioral activation, etc.) target each component of the problem. Clients are more likely to comply with treatment if they understand why particular techniques are being used.

In addition to presenting a model for maintenance and treatment of the problems focused on, other information can also be shared during psychoeducation. Clients are often interested to learn about prevalence rates and other related information about the problems they are having (e.g., average age of onset, rates in men versus women, etc.). Psychoeducation can also include some discussion of the etiology of the particular problem. In contrast to analytic therapies, where the goal is to understand what occurred in clients' lives to cause the problem, discussions of etiology in CBT are typically kept very general. For example, clients with anorexia and bulimia are often taught about the "multidetermined" nature of eating disorders (e.g., Garner, 1993). While some time can certainly be spent discussing how these general etiological models fit the client's own experiences, far less time is spent delving into these issues in CBT than in other forms of therapy.

Making Psychoeducation a Discussion

Psychoeducational material should not be delivered in lecture format when therapy is conducted with clients on an individual basis (some treatment programs do include group psychoeducation delivered in lecture format). Delivering the material as a lecture is a surefire way to damage rapport. Most clients have a great deal to say on the topic of their own psychological difficulties. It is usually frustrating for them to be fed all of this information without being given the opportunity to share how it applies to them. Similarly, the clinician misses out on crucial information that would be helpful in terms of case conceptualization and treatment planning. Clients come away from lecture sessions like this feeling misunderstood and seeing the clinician as a person who just likes to hear him- or herself speak.

Striking a balance between sharing information and keeping the client involved is particularly difficult for beginning clinicians. Some beginning clinicians become overly wedded to manuals, sometimes even memorizing certain passages in order to make sure that they deliver the information correctly. The end result, however, is often a rote presentation of material with no opportunity for clients to play a role.

How can this problem be ameliorated? Preparation is important. Clinicians must read more widely than just the treatment manual. They should have general knowledge of the kinds of difficulties that they are treating so that they can answer questions that are typically asked at this stage in therapy. Certainly this knowledge increases with time as you read more widely and gain more experience with clients, but even early on it is important to feel comfortable with "the basics."

Another general tip is to come with a rough outline for the psychoeducation session(s). We call this a "tip sheet." Its purpose is to cue you to cover each point. Tip sheets can also be used to remind clinicians to include clients in the discussion. You can put a big note to yourself at the top of the page ("Ask questions!") or make some notes on ways that each concept might apply to the client based on your case conceptualization (e.g., next to "family environment," the clinician could make a note that Michael mentioned during his assessment having grown up with a critical mother). These little notes can serve as cues for getting the client involved.

Some beginning clinicians worry that clients will see the tips as a cheat sheet and so perceive the clinician as incompetent. In our view, if the sheet is developed correctly, including only the bare-bones points (rather than detailed information), clients will rarely even notice that it is there. If clients do notice or even if they ask about it, it is unlikely that they will judge their clinician negatively because of it. Clinicians can simply say, "Oh, I always bring my list of points so that I make sure to cover all the important information with you." In other words, frame it as a benefit to the client, rather than as an anxiety-reducing strategy for you. Certainly, glancing down occasionally at notes is far superior to reading from detailed notes or directly from the manual or "winging it" and delivering information in a disorganized manner.

REVISITING THE CASE OF MICHAEL

The Hope et al. (2000) treatment manual provides a great deal of psychoeducational information that was shared with Michael. A sample "tip sheet" for covering this material is presented in Table 6.2. Michael and his therapist covered this material over the course of Sessions 1 and 2.

TABLE 6.2. Psychoeducational Material "Tip Sheet" for Michael

Session 1

1. Review diagnostic criteria for social phobia and discuss prevalence and other descriptives.

2. Discuss the distinction between "normal" and "problematic" social anxiety.

3. Introduce the three components of anxiety: physiological, cognitive, and behavioral.
   • With behavioral component, make sure to discuss role of avoidance in maintenance of disorder.
   • Use whiteboard to demonstrate downward spiral of anxiety.
   • Use whiteboard to demonstrate how various techniques used in treatment can break this cycle.

Session 2

4. Discuss possible causes of social anxiety.
   • Genetics
   • Family environment
   • Important experiences

   These can lead to development of . . .
   • Dysfunctional thinking patterns (including external locus of control; perfectionistic standards; and low self-efficacy)

   . . . which can play out in troublesome ways in actual situations . . .
   • Dysfunctional thinking → distraction → negative outcomes in social situations (e.g., forgetting what you are going to say).
   • Dysfunctional thinking → avoidance (not going into situation at all)

Treatment Session 1

As discussed earlier, the session had begun with the therapist's rough agenda, as shown in Table 6.1. The therapist and Michael had agreed during their feedback session to start therapy with a main focus on social phobia. Since they had already discussed the diagnostic criteria and prevalence of social phobia, the first treatment session began with just a brief review.

Michael and his clinician then discussed the difference between the social anxiety that is experienced at some time or another by most people versus the social anxiety that requires treatment. Based on their meetings thus far, Michael's clinician was concerned that he felt "silly" for seeking treatment for what he essentially saw as shyness. She wanted to emphasize to Michael that seeking help for his problems was not silly, since they were quite pervasive (e.g., they did not just happen from time to time) and were causing him a great deal of distress and impairment in functioning. The excessiveness of his anxiety, and the fact that his anxiety stood in the way of his doing many things indicated that he had social phobia, not just "normal" social anxiety. This discussion was not meant to make Michael feel worse about his lot in life, but rather to show him that it was perfectly appropriate for him to want to work on these significant problems.

Next, Michael's clinician introduced to him the concept of the "three components of anxiety"—the physiological component, the cognitive component, and the behavioral component. Michael was asked to describe how he experiences each of the components. Michael explained that when he feels anxious, his blushes quite badly, his voice shakes, and he sweats profusely (the physiological component). When they began to discuss the cognitive component, Michael said, "I know that when I am anxious, the thoughts come fast and furiously, but it is hard now to even think of all of them." His therapist was able to help him out a bit by referring back to her notes from their previous interactions—Michael reported thinking, "I always screw up," "They'll think I'm an idiot," and "Everyone notices how anxious I am." With physiological symptoms fresh in his mind, Michael added, "My face will be as red as a tomato," and "My voice will be so shaky no one will understand me."

With a good sense of Michael's cognitive symptoms, they then moved on to the behavioral component of anxiety, with the clinician asking Michael what he *does* in social situations to try to make himself feel less anxious. Michael reported that when giving speeches or answering questions in class, he tries to read verbatim from notes. When meeting new people, he tries to keep conversations as short as possible, so that there is less chance for him to "mess up." Michael was also asked about overt avoidance—things he will not do at all because of anxiety. In the year prior to presenting for treatment, he had found it quite difficult to avoid anything since so many activities were required of him at the seminary, like answering questions in class and leading religious services. Yet, when pressed, Michael admitted that he never volunteered to answer questions in class or to lead a service. He also reported that he never initiated conversations with women or with male superiors at work. In both of these cases, he would only speak if spoken to first, or in the case of his superiors, if he had a mandatory meeting.

At this point, the clinician helped Michael to see the advantages and disadvantages of avoidance through Socratic dialogue:

CLINICIAN: Among people with anxiety disorders, we see a lot of avoidance behaviors. Why do you think this is the case?

MICHAEL: Because it helps?

CLINICIAN: What do you mean, "it helps"?

MICHAEL: Well, it keeps the anxiety in check. If coffee and snacks are served after a meeting at the seminary, I am much more comfortable if I talk to the few guys that I am comfortable with than if I go right up to the Father Superior and talk to him.

CLINICIAN: So, in the short term, avoidance is a pretty good strategy?

MICHAEL: I think so. Do you?

CLINICIAN: I do, actually. But, there is another side to consider. What about in the long run?

MICHAEL: Not such a good strategy.

CLINICIAN: Why? Sounds like you could just feel calm forever by avoiding the situations that make you anxious.

MICHAEL: Well, it doesn't seem to work that way, does it?

CLINICIAN: What do you mean?

MICHAEL: It's landed me in therapy.

CLINICIAN: That's true. So, what do you think is so detrimental about avoidance?

MICHAEL: You never get over the things that make you nervous.

CLINICIAN: What would you need to do in order to get over it?

MICHAEL: I guess just do it and see that it isn't that bad.

CLINICIAN: That's right. That's where exposures come in—doing the frightening things and seeing that they aren't that bad.

MICHAEL: Right, I can see the point now.

CLINICIAN: That's good. It's an important point to think about. We're going to be talking some more about the approach to treatment next time, but before we do, I want to spend some time considering how these three components of anxiety fit together.

MICHAEL: Okay.

For the remainder of the first session of psychoeducation, Michael and his clinician considered the interaction of the physiological, the cognitive, and the behavioral components of anxiety. Using the template included in the Hope et al. (2000) manual (p. 25), Michael and his clinician mapped out on the whiteboard the "downward spiral of anxiety"— a visual depiction of how the physiological, cognitive, and behavioral components of anxiety interact to create missed opportunities and negative feelings. This is illustrated in Figure 6.1.

Working through such a figure can be quite demoralizing to clients. The end product demonstrates a vicious cycle, but does not address how

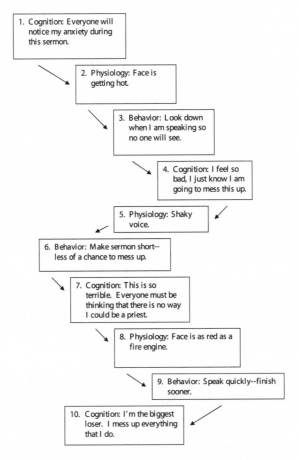

1. Cognition: Everyone will notice my anxiety during this sermon.

2. Physiology: Face is getting hot.

3. Behavior: Look down when I am speaking so no one will see.

4. Cognition: I feel so bad, I just know I am going to mess this up.

5. Physiology: Shaky voice.

6. Behavior: Make sermon short-- less of a chance to mess up.

7. Cognition: This is so terrible. Everyone must be thinking that there is no way I could be a priest.

8. Physiology: Face is as red as a fire engine.

9. Behavior: Speak quickly--finish sooner.

10. Cognition: I'm the biggest loser. I mess up everything that I do.

FIGURE 6.1. Michael's downward spiral of anxiety.

to break this cycle. In order to ensure that Michael left the session with a feeling of hopefulness, not hopelessness, his clinician explained that treatment would involve interrupting this vicious cycle before it got out of control and caused these missed opportunities and negative feelings. At this point, Michael asked a valuable question:

MICHAEL: But, with all that going on, how do you even know where to start?

CLINICIAN: Michael, that's a great question. Although it seems overwhelming to have these three processes going on all at once, it actually means that there are more ways to break the vicious cycle. You can "chip away" at it in various places.

MICHAEL: What do you mean?

CLINICIAN: Well, we have identified three components of anxiety, and we can really attack it in any of those areas.

MICHAEL: Oh, so if I think differently, that might help?

CLINICIAN: Right. And, changing your behaviors might help.

MICHAEL: How can I change the physiological stuff though? I've always blushed.

CLINICIAN: That's a good point . . . some of that is difficult to change, and some just naturally decreases as less anxiety is experienced in social situations. But, we can also change the way that you think about the symptoms. Remember, all of these components are related, so changing how you think about physical symptoms might make the physical symptoms less salient and important to you.

MICHAEL: What do you mean?

CLINICIAN: Well, through cognitive restructuring, we can explore how bad it is to blush.

MICHAEL: It's terrible.

CLINICIAN: Why?

MICHAEL: Because everyone sees.

CLINICIAN: That's possible. Or some people might notice and some might not. What's so bad about people noticing that you blush?

MICHAEL: They'll think I'm a loser.

CLINICIAN: All of them?

MICHAEL: What do you mean?

CLINICIAN: Every person that notices you blush will think you're a loser?

MICHAEL: Maybe not every single one.

CLINICIAN: Do you notice when people blush?

MICHAEL: Of course! I always feel so bad for people.

CLINICIAN: So, you don't think people who blush are losers?

MICHAEL: No, but some people might think that.

CLINICIAN: Some might think that. What would you think of them?

MICHAEL: Well, I guess it's pretty mean. Not a great way to judge people.

CLINICIAN: Tell me more about that.

MICHAEL: There must be more important grounds to judge people on, like if they are nice, and hard-working, and intelligent.

CLINICIAN: So, let me ask you—how much value would you place on the judgment of a person who thinks you're a loser because you blush?

MICHAEL: Not much. I can't see wanting to be friends with someone like that.

CLINICIAN: Okay . . . this was a quick example of using cognitive restructuring to examine thoughts about blushing, a physical symptom. I don't expect that after this brief conversation, you are no longer going to care about blushing. But, if we did a bit more work on this, what might happen to the symptom?

MICHAEL: Well, I might start noticing it less.

CLINICIAN: Would that impact your behavior?

MICHAEL: I might stop feeling like I need to look down or finish conversations so quickly.

CLINICIAN: And, any chance it could affect the actual blushing?

MICHAEL: Gee, I doubt it.

CLINICIAN: You could be right. It is possible that you blush easily. But, it is also possible that if you notice it less, you will be less anxious, and therefore you won't get as red as you might have if you noticed it and got very upset by it.

MICHAEL: I see what you're saying. By noticing and getting upset, I might actually make the blushing worse.

CLINICIAN: We can explore that in our time together. It's possible. The bottom line is just to keep in mind how changing thoughts and behaviors can have a very positive impact on physical symptoms of anxiety without actually trying to blush less, which can be very difficult.

MICHAEL: That makes a lot of sense.

At the end of therapy sessions, it can be very useful to have clients summarize what they have learned. Sometimes, it can be helpful to maintain a running list of "take-home messages" that clients can carry with them and glance at in difficult situations. Here is a look at the end of Michael's first therapy session:

CLINICIAN: So, Michael, the end of our session is just about here. Let's review what we discussed today before we finish up.

MICHAEL: Okay.

CLINICIAN: Did you find today's session helpful? What did you learn?

MICHAEL: Yes, it was definitely helpful and informative. I learned a lot.

CLINICIAN: What was the most helpful thing you learned?

MICHAEL: Avoidance is bad!

CLINICIAN: That's a good one. I often create with clients a list of "take-home messages" that they can carry around with them and look at in difficult situations. Would this be a good first item for the list?

MICHAEL: Absolutely. I can see that it could be helpful to remember that when I really want to avoid something.

CLINICIAN: Exactly—a helpful thought to keep in mind. What else did you learn today?

MICHAEL: I know I learned a lot, but that is the thing that's sticking in my head the most.

CLINICIAN: Okay. That's great. To me, the real point of this session is to provide us with a framework for understanding why anxiety sticks around over time and how we can break into this vicious cycle of anxiety to make things easier for you. This really structures the therapy for us.

MICHAEL: Yeah, I like that idea that there are various ways to work on the problem.

CLINICIAN: Exactly. And, I think you'll really start to recognize how they are all related. Making a behavioral change, for example, can really change your thoughts. We are going to learn to be really aware of these connections between thoughts and behaviors. Actually, you can start working on this for homework this week.

MICHAEL: Homework?

CLINICIAN: I know you have a fair bit of that from school right now, but it's really important to work on your social anxiety every day, not just in the 1 hour each week when you are here. Like anything else, the more you put into the treatment, the more you will get out of it.

MICHAEL: Makes sense. So, what's the assignment?

CLINICIAN: During the week, I want you to make some notes about a few situations in which you experience social anxiety. What events do you have coming up this week where you expect to feel anxious?

MICHAEL: I have class almost every day. And I am leading a service at a nursing home on Sunday morning.

CLINICIAN: Great. Those sound like good situations to keep track of. What I'd like you to do is record a brief description of the event that brought on the anxiety, what physiological symptoms you experienced, what behaviors you engaged in, and what your thoughts were. This will help us to really understand how the three components of anxiety fit together in a variety of different situations.

MICHAEL: And you're going to look at my notes next week? Can I just tell you what happened instead of actually bringing in notes?

CLINICIAN: Why do you ask?

MICHAEL: Well, I'm not a great speller. And, writing isn't my strong suit. You know what they say about doctors!

CLINICIAN: Sounds like some anxiety talking.

MICHAEL: You'll just think I'm an idiot.

CLINICIAN: This comes up a lot with socially anxious clients. They worry that I will judge them negatively, just like they think others do. Let me reassure you that I am here to help you, and not to judge you. I don't care about spelling, and if I don't understand something you wrote, I'll just ask.

MICHAEL: So, I can't avoid writing down the homework?

CLINICIAN: Well, you tell me . . . what would be bad about this?

MICHAEL: It would feel good in the short run but probably mess something up in the long run.

CLINICIAN: Mess what up?

MICHAEL: Well, if you are telling me to write it, it must be for a reason.

CLINICIAN: It is. We want to see what you experience "in the moment." Sometimes, when we look back on something, it is hard to say what we were thinking, feeling, and doing. Writing down your observations in the moment is the best way to capture the experience of anxiety.

MICHAEL: I can see that. Sure, I'll do it.

The final "must-do" of every session is to ask clients if they have any questions or concerns. Right from the start of therapy, the tone should be set that questions and feedback are not only permitted, but actually encouraged. Again, this establishes the tone of collaborative empiricism that is so important in CBT.

Treatment Session 2

Michael returned to the clinic 1 week later for his second session of therapy. The agenda for this session was to finish the psychoeducational material and to design the hierarchy of feared situations. The session began with Michael giving a brief account of his week, a review of the homework assignment, and agenda setting for the remainder of the session. Michael had completed his homework, but, as had been predicted in the case conceptualization and at the end of the first session, his anxiety got in the way to some degree. Michael had typed his monitoring charts and when asked if he had spent a lot of time doing them, he admitted that he had done them quite efficiently throughout the week, but then spent hours the night before redoing them so that they would "look and sound okay." Michael's clinician reassured him that this was not necessary—quick notes from each situation would be fine—and that they could start to view his homework as an opportunity to test out his beliefs about needing to be perfect. His clinician encouraged him to do the homework more quickly in the upcoming week and test out his beliefs that (1) he would be judged negatively for a "shoddy" job and (2) they would not be as beneficial to the therapy process as if he did them more "perfectly." Michael agreed to try this out.

In the second session, the psychoeducation included a discussion of the possible causes of social anxiety. In Table 6.2 (see p. 114), we include a summary of the material that was covered with Michael. Although Michael's clinician presented all of this material to him, she did not spend a great deal of time on points that were not relevant to him. Given that she had done an initial case conceptualization, she had an idea of what points Michael would identify with, and as she presented the material she was able to reflect back on their earlier discussions. For example, since they had discussed Michael's family environment a fair bit, as the clinician presented this point she was able to say "We talked earlier about the important role that your family environment seems to have played in the development of your social anxiety. Let's spend a little bit more time now discussing that." At this prompting, Michael went on to explain that he had grown up in a family where impressions were very important. He recalled his mother kicking him under the table at family get-togethers if he started to say something "stupid." Prior to family functions or church events, Michael's mother would review specific rules for behavior with him and his sister. She would emphasize the importance of "perfect" table manners, not speaking to adults unless spoken to, and making sure one's appearance was neat and clean. Michael reported that he could not recall a time in his life when he was not concerned with the impressions of others.

Michael also remembered being teased in school for the physical symptoms of anxiety that he exhibited. As early as the first grade, Michael could remember other children calling him "tomato face." He explained that he started looking down as he spoke to others so that they would not notice his red face. He also recounted taking off heavy sweaters and wearing just a short-sleeve shirt at school during the winter so that he would make sure he did not turn too red. These habits of looking down and wearing lightweight clothes persisted to this day.

Michael also related to the idea that these early experiences might have contributed to the development of dysfunctional thinking patterns, particularly that of having perfectionistic standards for himself. Michael's therapist asked him how these dysfunctional thinking patterns played out in actual social situations.

CLINICIAN: When you're in a social situation, what is the impact of thinking how important it is to perform perfectly?

MICHAEL: Before I came here, I would have said, "It helps me to do a good job. If I wasn't thinking about it, I'd mess up even more." But I think I am catching on. If all I am thinking of is how important it is to be perfect, it might actually make me mess up because I am not paying attention.

CLINICIAN: That's a great observation. Any other problems with focusing on performing perfectly?

MICHAEL: Well, I seem to set myself up for failure. I guess I can accept that everyone makes mistakes sometimes, but I don't seem to allow this for myself.

CLINICIAN: So, when you leave a situation, how do you feel?

MICHAEL: Terrible. Always!

CLINICIAN: Does this have an impact on the next time you have to go into a similar situation?

MICHAEL: Sure. I go in assuming I will mess up, just like every other time.

CLINICIAN: That's a rough position to be in, isn't it?

MICHAEL: Yeah. I'm kind of my own worst enemy, aren't I?

CLINICIAN: Could be. We'll definitely spend some time thinking about that in our time together.

At this point, Michael's clinician summarized some of the factors that might have contributed to the development and subsequent maintenance of his social anxiety. They then reviewed the different aspects of the treatment program, drawing on all the material covered to this point. His therapist described systematic graduated exposure, cognitive restructuring, and homework, highlighting how each component of treatment would help with the problematic thinking and avoidance behaviors in which Michael was engaging.

CLINICIAN: This therapy includes three key components: systematic graduated exposure, cognitive restructuring, and homework. I know we've talked about all of these a bit during our time together, but let's just review them and see how they might help some of the problems we've been discussing.

MICHAEL: Okay.

CLINICIAN: We've talked some about exposures. These are behavioral exercises that involve confronting feared social situations. Now, what do we mean by "graduated" exposure?

MICHAEL: Thankfully, that we do them gradually.

CLINICIAN: Right, later in the session today, we are going to develop a hierarchy of feared situations, rank-ordered from least to most anxiety-provoking. We are going to work through them in that order so that you can use your earlier successes to help you out with the more difficult tasks. What do you think is the point of doing these exposures?

MICHAEL: Torturing me?

CLINICIAN: Well, I hope not! Any other thoughts?

MICHAEL: To show me that it's not that bad?

CLINICIAN: That's right. There's a few pieces to that. First, the longer you stay in a situation, the less anxious you'll get. And the more times you go into that same situation, the less anxious you'll be. We call this process "habituation." The basic idea is for you to learn that the anxiety will not stick around forever. The other goal with exposures is for you to be able to test out your beliefs.

MICHAEL: Like what you were saying about doing a sermon without any practice?

CLINICIAN: Right. And, besides torture, what would be the point of that?

MICHAEL: Well, I know what you want me to say. You want me to say that I would see that it wouldn't be as disastrous as I expect.

CLINICIAN: Right. And, by the way, I appreciate you pointing out that you and I are seeing things a bit differently here. I do believe that it would not be a complete disaster if you did a sermon without much practice. I know that you don't believe this right now. That's perfectly fine. The idea is to be open-minded enough to try things in different ways and see for yourself.

MICHAEL: Hard to imagine I could do it, but I do trust that it might get easier as we work on some other things.

CLINICIAN: That's the idea. Now, how about cognitive restructuring. What's that all about?

MICHAEL: Examining my thoughts?

CLINICIAN: Right. Cognitive restructuring allows you to analyze what you're thinking when you're anxious. We don't expect you to turn all your thoughts rosy and positive, but rather just to look at the thoughts more objectively and see if they make sense or if they are helpful. Now, remember how we discussed the relationship between thoughts and behaviors? How might cognitive restructuring impact behaviors?

MICHAEL: Well, if I think differently about things, I might be more willing to do them.

CLINICIAN: Right, and maybe even have some positive experiences in these situations.

MICHAEL: That would be nice.

CLINICIAN: How about what you said before about the effects of focusing on perfectionistic thoughts in social situations?

MICHAEL: It gets in the way.

CLINICIAN: So, if we changed around the thoughts a bit to be more accurate, what effect might that have?

MICHAEL: I might be able to focus better.

CLINICIAN: That would be great, wouldn't it?

MICHAEL: Sure.

CLINICIAN: So let's give some attention for a moment to the third component of treatment: homework. This is really important, as we discussed last week.

MICHAEL: Right, the more I put in, the more I get out.

CLINICIAN: Exactly. Let me just give you a sense of what kinds of homework I'll be assigning. You'll be doing a fair bit of monitoring, kind of like what you did this week, keeping track of your experiences in social situations. Once we start doing cognitive restructuring, I'll ask you to do some of that for homework. Also, while we'll be doing a lot of exposures here, doing them out there in your own environment will also be really important.

MICHAEL: That's going to be the hardest.

CLINICIAN: It is going to be hard, but by the time you start to do exposures, you'll have a lot of tools to help you out, like the ability to examine your thoughts in a more accurate and adaptive way. You'll be able to try out a lot of things here first, which can be really helpful.

MICHAEL: I'll have to trust you on that one.

CLINICIAN: Fair enough. Before we move on with our hierarchy, let's give a bit of thought to how you can get the most out of your time in treatment. What do you think would make your time here most worthwhile?

MICHAEL: Well, even though the idea of exposures terrifies me, I can see how the more you do, the easier it will probably get.

CLINICIAN: Right. Practice, practice, practice! It is also important to persevere. When things are hard, people have a tendency to give up, or to try something once and think it is too hard to do again. In this program, we encourage you to persevere—try things many times and know that with time, they will get easier.

MICHAEL: That's a good tip.

CLINICIAN: On that topic, how about perfectionistic standards? Is it okay to have perfectionistic standards about treatment?

MICHAEL: I suppose not.

CLINICIAN: Why?

MICHAEL: Because then I'd be setting myself up for failure even in treatment. That would be pretty stupid.

CLINICIAN: I don't know about it being stupid. It is reasonable that you would regard treatment as you regard other activities in your life. But I agree that having overly high standards for treatment could set you up for feeling like you are failing. We will come up with ways for you to catch yourself when you're beating yourself up, and then learn to give yourself credit for the hard work you're going to do.

MICHAEL: I could use tips like that.

CLINICIAN: Good. The final point I want to make is that people do well in treatment when they are willing to try new ways of doing things. When people come for treatment, it is generally because their current methods of dealing with anxiety aren't working. So, it is great to be open to doing things in new ways and seeing how it goes.

MICHAEL: I'm game. This social anxiety is getting in the way so much for me. . . . I really want to try to get over it.

CLINICIAN: I think we'll make a good team.

In the remaining time left in Session 2, Michael and his clinician developed a fear and avoidance hierarchy to guide the exposure component of treatment. This hierarchy was a list of social situations that Michael either completely avoided or that he did enter, but in which he experienced a great deal of anxiety. Each situation was rated using a 0–100 Subjective Units of Discomfort Scale (SUDS), where 0 represented no anxiety at all and 100 represented the most severe social anxiety Michael could imagine. The items in the hierarchy were rank ordered according to these anxiety ratings from least to most anxiety-provoking.

Because Michael and his clinician had already spent a fair bit of time together, and Michael had given a lot of thought to his problems with social anxiety, coming up with items for the hierarchy was quite easy. If clients are not as able to generate items as Michael was, a good strategy is to look back at the client's initial assessment. Often, measures would have been administered that would tap into specific situations or triggers that should be targeted during treatment. A copy of Michael's hierarchy is included in Figure 6.2. Michael suggested a number of items, and his clinician suggested a few more that Michael had mentioned over their last few meetings. The lowest item on Michael's hierarchy was rated a 50. He noted that there were many other

Item	SUDS
Doing a sermon without preparing	95
Doing a sermon for a large (100 + people) group	90
Speaking up at a meeting	85
Having a one-on-one conversation with a woman	80
Speaking to superiors	80
Being called on in class	80
Doing a sermon for a small group	80
Volunteering to answer a question in class if not sure of the answer	75
Speaking to a group of women in a work setting (e.g., nuns at community service project)	70
Interacting after church with parishioners	65
Having lunch with a group of classmates	60
Volunteering to answer a question in class if sure of answer	60
Having lunch with one classmate	50
Having a one-on-one conversation with a stranger (man)	50

FIGURE 6.2. Michael's hierarchy.

social situations he engaged in on a daily basis that elicited SUDS ratings of less than 50 (e.g., visiting parishioners at the hospital, chatting for a few minutes before class with his classmates). Since he was regularly doing these things, and not engaging in any subtle avoidance behaviors while doing so, they were not placed on his hierarchy. Rather, the lowest item on the hierarchy was a situation Michael was currently avoiding, but that he thought he would be able to confront quite early in treatment. In general, the low items on the hierarchy (regardless of their numerical rating) should be things that clients would be able to successfully confront early in treatment with a moderate (but manageable) amount of anxiety.

Michael was given a copy of his hierarchy to take home at the end of the session and was invited to add any new items he thought of. He was also told to continue monitoring the three components of anxiety, as he had done during the previous week. At the close of the session, Michael was invited to ask questions and was asked what he had learned during the session. Michael came up with two "take-home messages" to add to his list: "I am probably my own worst enemy" and "Paying attention to doing a perfect job might actually make me do a bad job."

This brings us to the close of Michael's first two therapy sessions. A summary of key points to keep in mind for the first few sessions of therapy are included in Table 6.3.

BEFORE MOVING ON: A NOTE ON HOMEWORK IN CBT

Before moving on to the next stage of therapy, let's give some consideration to the use of homework in CBT. With Michael, homework was assigned starting after the first session of therapy. This is typical in CBT, emphasizing from the start that it is an active approach to treatment in which clients play a central role.

It is important that clients understand *why* they are being asked to do homework. One compelling reason is that, at least for some kinds of difficulties, homework compliance has been related to treatment outcome. Why might this be the case? There are a number of potential reasons, all of which can be shared with clients. Again, Socratic questioning can be used to help clients derive their own hypotheses as to why homework might be helpful. Homework affords greater opportunity to practice new skills than just coming to therapy once per week. Furthermore, homework allows clients to practice these skills in the "real world." Work done outside of sessions can actually hold more weight for clients than work done in sessions. During sessions, clients often discount their accomplishments. Doing some good work in session might be attributed to the guidance of a supportive clinician or to a "safe" environment.

TABLE 6.3. Tips to Remember in the First Few Sessions of Therapy

- Come prepared—review the case, devise a treatment plan, set session-by-session agendas, prepare a "cheat sheet" for psychoeducational material.
- At the beginning of the first session, review presenting problems, ask the client if anything has changed since his or her assessment, and inquire about expectancies for treatment.
- When describing treatment and doing psychoeducation, use Socratic questioning to keep the client engaged, rather than lapsing into lecture format.
- Welcome questions from the client about key concepts.
- Appreciate that the client does not have to "buy" all the concepts or be 100% sure that treatment will help. Rather, infuse the client with the spirit of empiricism—make sure he or she is open to try new things and see for him- or herself the effects of doing so.
- Introduce homework, and discuss its importance, early in treatment.
- Discuss with the client what he or she can do to increase the likelihood that treatment will help.

When clients try things out on their own and see positive results in their own environments, they often feel a burst of confidence—not only in themselves, but also in the core techniques that have been taught in therapy. This helps clients to see that they will be able to continue serving as their own clinicians once therapy is over. In Chapter 9, we speak more to the very important issue of homework compliance.

Chapter 7

■ ■ ■

DEALING WITH INITIAL CHALLENGES IN COGNITIVE-BEHAVIORAL THERAPY

It this chapter, we begin by discussing some challenges that quite often present themselves in the early stages of CBT. Early in treatment, it is essential that clients understand and accept the CBT approach—when they do not, progressing with the treatment can be difficult and frustrating for both the client and clinician. We discuss why some clients have a hard time with the approach and how to move them along so that they can best engage in the treatment. In the latter portion of the chapter, we focus on a particularly stressful clinical challenge—working with suicidal clients. We discuss how to assess risk for suicide and how to best deal with clients at this very difficult time. Finally, we look at some challenges that clinicians themselves bring to the table that can have an important impact on the course of therapy.

CHALLENGES IN SOCIALIZING CLIENTS TO CBT

Starting the CBT process is a crucial stage in therapy. It is essential to get clients "on board" with the CBT approach to understanding and treating psychological difficulties. Early in therapy, clients should feel some sense of hope for the future. They should believe that they are going to acquire knowledge and skills that will lead to better functioning. If clients are dissatisfied or have doubts early in the therapy process, these problems should be handled promptly.

"My Client Is Unhappy with the Pace of Therapy"

Some therapy protocols jump into active work right away, perhaps doing a behavioral exercise or some cognitive restructuring in the very first session. Other protocols include a bit more time for "buildup," sometimes including a few sessions that are quite didactic in nature. While it is good practice to get clients involved in psychoeducation, there is no doubt that some clients wonder at this stage of therapy when they are going to start working on their "real problems."

There are a few ways to deal with this. First, it is important to gauge clients' levels of understanding. For clients who catch on to concepts quickly, it is appropriate to move a little more quickly through introductory material and get on to the "meat" of the therapy. This is not to say that the material should not be covered well. Rather, progress at a pace that seems comfortable for the client. In some cases, you will be concerned that the client does not understand the core concepts, yet still expresses the desire to move on. This is tricky. Some clients will understand the concepts best by *doing*; for these clients, progressing on to a more active part of the therapy might be fine. However, we always want to ensure that clients understand the rationale for *why* we do certain things. They do not need to *believe* the rationale (e.g., if you stop doing compulsions during OCD treatment, feared outcomes are unlikely to occur), but they do need to understand the purpose of each therapy technique (e.g, refraining from compulsions should help me to see whether or not my feared consequences will occur) and be open to trying them. A clear understanding of the cognitive-behavioral model for treating difficulties serves as the scaffolding, or support, for the treatment.

"My Client Is Having Difficulties with the CBT Approach"

You have explained CBT to your client and ensured that she understands the approach. Although she has a clear understanding, she is doubtful that CBT will work for her. You encourage her to give it a try, so she agrees to do some behavioral experiments and some cognitive restructuring. From an objective point of view, all is going well. Yet, the client continues to discount the approach and remains steadfast in her conviction that it will not work for her. What can you do?

When clients remain convinced that CBT will not work for them, despite having some objectively positive experiences with it, there are several explanations to consider. First, clients might reject the CBT approach as a means of resisting change. Sometimes CBT does not match clients' beliefs about the etiology of their difficulties. If clients do not see their difficulties as being caused by faulty cognitions and dysfunctional behaviors, they might have a hard time accepting that change can be accomplished by changing cognitions and behaviors. There are two kinds of mismatches between clients' etiological beliefs and using CBT as a means to treat their difficulties.

"My Client Believes That It Is Necessary to Delve into the Past to 'Get Better'"

Some clients will wonder whether CBT will "work" given that it does not involve an extensive exploration into early experiences that might have led to clients' current difficulties. This type of concern is often based on misconceptions that clients have about CBT. Many clients (and indeed other mental health professionals, too) think that CBT completely ignores the past. This is not true. Clinicians who do CBT are most definitely interested in the connection between past experiences and current beliefs and behaviors. This is perhaps best exhibited through our interest in core beliefs, which are thought to develop during childhood and underlie psychological problems.

There are many advantages to spending some time with clients exploring connections between past experiences and current beliefs and behaviors. Most notably, such explorations can help clients to consider whether other factors played a role in their difficulties besides their own shortcomings. Rather than assigning blame solely to themselves, they can begin to see how other factors might have contributed to the development of problematic thoughts and behaviors. Identifying these factors can then shed light on what can be done to ameliorate these problems.

Take, for example, a 20-year-old client with an eating disorder. By exploring the origins of her excessive concern with shape and weight, the therapist learned the following information from the client: (1) She grew up in a home with a mother who dieted and was excessively concerned with her own shape and weight and that of her daughter; (2) throughout her childhood and adolescence she attended a school for the arts and majored in dance, thus facing undue pressure at school as well to be thin; (3) she recently stopped dancing and felt at a complete loss for what to do with her life. Knowing such information is greatly helpful for conceptualizing the case. It suggests that the client grew up in an environment where value was *only* placed on shape and weight, to the exclusion of any other attributes like intelligence or kindness to others. This value system was reinforced throughout her childhood and adolescence not only at home, but also in school by her teachers and her peer group. It made perfect sense to the therapist that a young woman growing up in this environment would be at risk for developing problems with eating and he communicated this to the client.

Where CBT diverges from other schools of therapy is that it does not exclusively dwell in the past. Once the case is clearly conceptualized, CBT techniques are used to change *current* problematic thoughts and behaviors. Again, this does not mean that the past is ignored. The role of past experiences is considered throughout treatment, particularly in relation to the development of core beliefs. However, simply understanding the origins of the problem is not thought to be the panacea. Rather, the client must take this knowledge and use it to change the dysfunctional beliefs and behaviors that are maintaining current problems. In the case of the client with the eating disorder, treatment might entail helping her to explore other career paths besides dancing, developing new skills and hobbies that tap into other talents and interests, working on skills for better communication with her mother, expanding her social group beyond the world of dancing to include people who put value on other attributes besides shape and weight, and, of course, learning healthier eating and exercise behaviors. Once clients understand that the past will not be ignored in CBT, and that CBT is an effective treatment despite not focusing exclusively on the past, these concerns will often be quelled.

"My Client Thinks His Problems Are Biologically Determined"

Another belief system that can interfere in CBT (or in any psychotherapy, for that matter) is the belief that psychological difficulties are solely attributable to biological factors. It seems odd that clients who hold this etiological belief would come to psychotherapy, but they do from time to time, and the nature of their attributions can interfere in their progress.

A good place to start with these clients is with some psychoeducation about the relative roles played by both biology and environment in the development and maintenance of psychological disorders. There is ample evidence to suggest that both biological and psychological factors play a role in the etiology and maintenance of most, if not all, psychological problems. It is not surprising then that many problems seem equally amenable to psychotherapy and medication. Interestingly, even CBT alone (e.g., without medication) can impact biology. Studies have shown that CBT alters brain function in much the same way as psychotropic medications (e.g., see Furmark et al., 2002; Goldapple et al., 2004).

It is also prudent to delve into the reasons why clients are resistant to attributing their difficulties to psychological factors. It is here that cognitive work can be very effective. Ask your client what it means to him or her to be "mentally ill" or "depressed" or "bulimic." Often clients will reveal all sorts of self-deprecatory thoughts associated with their difficulties, and some will even tell you that thinking of their problems as being caused by biology alone is simply "easier." These kinds of thoughts are legitimate targets for cognitive restructuring.

SPECIAL CONSIDERATIONS FOR CLIENTS TAKING MEDICATION WHILE DOING CBT

Many patients will be able to share in our belief that both psychological and physiological factors might contribute to the difficulties that they are having and that it may make sense to do CBT and take medication concurrently. While this decision is by no means problematic, it can be associated with various dilemmas, both in terms of the role that should be played by the nonprescribing mental health practitioner, as well as the way that clients interpret positive changes that they make.

Sharing Our Expertise

Whenever we treat clients who are also on medication, it is essential that we be in touch with the prescribing physician and work together to coordinate our treatment efforts. There are numerous reasons why this coordination is so essential to our clients' care. Although cognitive-behavioral clinicians are not experts in pharmacotherapy, most know (or should know) about psychiatric medications that are typically prescribed, which medications are indicated for which conditions, and which doses are proper for which conditions. It is interesting to note that the majority of prescriptions for psychotropic drugs are not written by psychiatrists. For instance, a recent study found that 85% of prescriptions for antidepressants were written by general practitioners, while only 11% were written by psychiatrists (McManus et al., 2000). Although some nonpsychiatrists have extensive knowledge about mental health, general practitioners and other prescribing physicians take care of innumerable health problems, and it should not come as a surprise that we sometimes find fault in their diagnostic or treatment decisions.

This emphasizes the importance of having contact with your clients' prescribing physician. At times there might not be a great deal to discuss beyond simply touching base and agreeing to be in contact if particular issues arise (e.g., a client wanting to discontinue medication sometime during the course of therapy). At other times, you might want to discuss with physicians their choice of medications and their decisions about dose. Some beginning clinicians worry that by doing this they will be perceived by physicians as being confrontational or critical. In fact, many physicians, particularly those with less expertise in mental health, feel quite positive about establishing a collaborative relationship with a clinician. If, however, you or your client finds the prescribing physician unwilling to consider alternatives (or if a client's case is very complex), it might be best to refer the client to a physician who has expertise with psychotropic drugs and the treatment of psychological disorders.

Another thing to keep in mind is that many of your clients' concerns about medication might actually be shared with you, rather than their prescribing physician, because clients will see you more frequently and will likely feel somewhat closer to you. You may not be able to answer all of your clients' questions (nor should you answer all of them, such as questions about adjusting dosages, etc.), but you can certainly be of some help. For example, some psychiatric medications may cause clients to experience increased anxiety when they first start to take them. You can help the client to realize that this is a normal experience and that this side effect should diminish with time. Similarly, some medications do not have their desired effect for a few weeks. In these circumstances, the clinician should encourage clients to remain compliant and give the medication some time to work. It is also good practice to check in with clients about side effects on occasion. Some might be embarrassing to talk about (e.g., difficulties with sexual functioning), and clients may appreciate your bringing them up and making clear that these difficulties are quite common.

Making Sure That Medication Does Not Interfere in the Process of CBT

Another time to contact the prescribing physician is when the medication regimen is having a negative impact on the CBT. We sometimes see clients on so many medications or on such high doses that they can barely stay awake through sessions, much less do work on their own between sessions. Medication can also interfere with certain treatment techniques, for example, imaginal or *in vivo* exposure. When confronting feared situations, it is essential that clients actually experience fear. In this way, clients will learn that anxiety habituates over time and that they can manage in situations that cause them distress. Medications that block the fear response (e.g., benzodiazepines) may interfere with clients' opportunity to benefit from this learning experience. For treatment programs that involve a large exposure component, it is best to talk with the prescribing physician about discontinuing anxiolytic medication, or at the least instructing clients to take them at a time when they will not interfere with in-session work or homework.

The Issue of Medication and Attributions for Change

When clients take medication and participate in CBT at the same time, attention must be paid to the clients' attributions for therapy success and failure. When clients make improvements, do they attribute them to their own efforts in CBT or to taking medication each day? The response to this question can have a major impact on maintenance of treatment gains.

Consider a client with social phobia. This client had been on medication and in different kinds of therapy for many years with no improvement in his symptoms. He enrolled in group treatment for social phobia and began to experience significant changes in the way that he thought about and behaved in social situations. About midway through the group treatment, we remarked on how well the client was doing and asked him to what he attributed his successes. The client (in a very convincing voice) said, "It's my medication. It's *finally* started to work."

Interestingly, this client had been on medication for years with no change in his symptoms. Furthermore, over the past number of weeks, he had been making a great deal of effort, putting himself in social situations that he had avoided for years. To the objective reader, this pattern of attributions might seem silly, but to the client it seemed completely sensible. Clinicians should be concerned that clients like this might be at risk for relapse once therapy is over (as was indeed shown in one study with clients who were treated for panic disorder; see Basoglu, Marks, Kilic, Brewin, & Swinson, 1994). Although our client's gains clearly appeared to be attributable to the new skills that he learned in the group and to all of his hard work, he did not recognize this, and, therefore, he might have failed to continue to apply these skills once therapy ended.

It is important to explore these issues with CBT clients who are also taking medication. If a client is showing improvement, ask him or her to what he or she attributes these changes (as we did with our client). If there is evidence of faulty thinking, engage in some cognitive restructuring to get clients to the point of seeing that their hard work with CB techniques must have played at least some part in the positive changes that they have made. This might also be a good time to talk further to clients about the long-term efficacy of CBT. CBT has better "staying power" than medications, presumably because clients learn new skills that they can continue to use in their daily lives once formal treatment ends.

Helping Clients to Discontinue Medication

Sometimes clients come to therapy on medication, having been told by their physicians that they must be on it in order to manage the difficulties that they are having. Other clients might have decided more freely to go on medication, but do not want to continue to take it indefinitely. Still others may come upon life events, such as pregnancy, that make it difficult or unsafe for them to continue taking medications with which they might otherwise be satisfied. These clients see psychotherapy as a way to learn skills that will permit them to come off the medication and manage their difficulties on their own. For clients who have been told that medication is their only option, it is our job to inform them otherwise. Though it is typically inappropriate to criticize the use of medication, it is very important that clients learn that CBT is also a very effective approach to treatment—and a very effective stand-alone approach to treatment. Clients are often thrilled to learn this.

It is not our job to advise clients on how to discontinue medication, but we can certainly work together in a coordinated manner with the prescribing physician. It can be very beneficial for clients to discontinue their medication while they are still in therapy so that they can have some help dealing with their anxiety around doing so and with the possible return of symptoms.

SPECIAL CHALLENGES: WORKING WITH SUICIDAL CLIENTS

The clinical challenges described thus far come up frequently in our work as CBT therapists. A less frequent, but more stressful, clinical challenge is working with clients who are suicidal. Even for experienced clinicians, dealing with suicidal clients is a nerve-wracking experience. For less experienced clinicians, the fears are likely to be significant, driven by not knowing how to assess risk in order to protect the client and oneself. We try here to impart some knowledge so that clinicians can focus on helping suicidal clients, rather than getting lost in their own anxieties.

The Legalities

There are three cardinal administrative rules to follow when dealing with suicidal clients, which benefit your client, but also protect you. First, document everything. Second, seek out supervision. Third, consult with colleagues.

Document Everything

It is essential to keep clear records all the time, but even more so when dealing with suicidal clients. As you speak to the client, try to record direct quotations (e.g., "I'm feeling at my absolute lowest ever, but I can't do anything to myself because of my kids"). After meeting with the client, write a thorough note. Describe the client's complaint, the nature of your assessment, and the actions taken to reduce risk (e.g., making a contract, providing the client with emergency numbers, asking about social support, etc.). Any subsequent contact with the client should also be recorded (e.g., phone calls).

Seek Supervision

For the beginning clinician, the next cardinal rule is to seek supervision. Beginning clinicians are often concerned about being perceived by their supervisors as lacking independence or good clinical skills. They also do not want to be perceived by their clients as lacking experience. This is a time to put those concerns away. If, in the midst of the assessment, you are feeling unsure of yourself, get backup. If you have managed the assessment on your own, consult with a supervisor before implementing a course of action. Ultimately, your supervisor is responsible for the client's welfare. Be sure that your supervisor signs off on your chart notes to indicate that he or she agreed with the decisions that you have made.

Consult with Colleagues

The final cardinal rule, which pertains regardless of your level of experience, is to consult with your colleagues. When faced with any ethical/legal dilemma, it is best to consult with colleagues and gain some consensus on the "right" course of action. Consultations with colleagues should also be recorded in the client's record.

WHAT SKILLS AND KNOWLEDGE DO YOU NEED TO ASSESS SUICIDE RISK?

Every clinician will be faced, numerous times in their careers, with clients who say that they think they would be better off dead. The moment we hear such a phrase, however, it would be inappropriate to immediately send the client to the hospital. Rather, time must be spent to understand the meaning behind these words and decide on the best course of action to take.

Be Mindful of Your Reactions

The first thing to keep in mind when faced with these words is to be mindful of your emotional reaction. It is very important to make it clear to the client that he or she can share this information with you. Do your best to accept this communication with the same serious attentiveness that you would convey at any other time. Maintain the same tone that you were using prior to receiving this information—remain calm, attentive, and nonjudgmental. It is also very important to try to normalize the client's experience. Again, we do not want to discount the importance of suicidal thoughts. However, clients are often very ashamed of them, and we do not want that shame to stand in the way of their being honest and, in turn, getting the help that they need. A good response might be "It must have been really difficult for you to have shared this with me. I know that it's really scary to have those kinds of thoughts. A lot of people, at one time or another, do have thoughts about suicide. Let's talk a bit more about this and try to figure out what we can do help you out."

Come Armed with Knowledge

With the proper tone set, the task at hand is to assess the client's risk for suicide. Knowing who is at risk is not an exact science. The base rate of suicide is very low in the general population and even in psychiatric populations—even though the risk is about 5 times higher than in the general population. This low base rate of occurrences makes research into risk factors difficult. Furthermore, many researchers are "scared away" from doing research on suicidal clients. The liability in these litigious times is just too great. This is unfortunate, since arming ourselves with empirical data is the best way to help our clients. With these caveats, let us consider what we do know.

Although we are unable here to review all the literature on suicide, we have found Rudd and Joiner's (1998; see also Cukrowicz, Wingate, Driscoll, & Joiner, 2004; Joiner, Walker, Rudd, & Jobes, 1999) model for suicide risk particularly helpful. They have suggested that there are predisposing factors, risk factors, and protective factors for attempted and completed suicide. We review these factors here, and provide in Table 7.1 a summary of questions that you can ask clients who are suicidal.

Predisposing Factors

Predisposing factors are those that are long-standing and unchangeable. For example, genetics and other biological factors (e.g., low or unstable levels of serotonin) may play a role. Other predisposing factors that have been associated with suicide risk are a chaotic family history (e.g., separation and/or divorce in the family of origin, numerous changes in residence, parental psychopathology, etc.) and a history of physical or sexual abuse. It is important to keep in mind that although these factors may predispose an individual to attempt suicide, these factors do not guarantee that a person ever will attempt suicide. Neither does their absence assure that the person will not attempt suicide.

TABLE 7.1. Suicide Risk Assessment Questions

- How long have you been thinking about suicide? When you think about suicide, what kinds of thoughts do you have? (*Be attuned to a hopeless state of mind— the general belief that one's lot in life is unchanging and that one exhibits little control over outcomes in one's life.*)

- What has been going on in your life lately? Has anything specific gone on in the past 6 months that has made you contemplate suicide? (*Life events to inquire about: breakup of relationship, other interpersonal losses, interpersonal conflicts [including abusive relationships], loss of job, legal difficulties, etc.*)

- Have you made any plans for how you would attempt suicide? (*Things to consider: How lethal is the plan? Is it specific, detailed, and well planned? Does the individual have the means to carry it out [e.g., if he or she plans to commit suicide with a gun, does he or she have access to one?]? Does the person seem to have the "courage" to carry out the plan?*)

- Have you attempted suicide before? By what means? How have you been doing since that attempt?

- Have you done anything else in the past to harm yourself, like taking pills or cutting yourself?

- Do you have any social support? Do you live alone or with someone else? Do you have any children?

- What are your thoughts about the future? Do you have any hope that things could change for you? If there anything or anyone (e.g., children) making you want to hang on?

Other questions for the clinician to consider:

- Does the client currently meet criteria for a specific psychiatric diagnosis? (*Consider both Axis I and Axis II diagnoses.*)

- Does the client seem to be impulsive, or does he or she seem to be a methodical problem solver with good self-control?

- Does the client have a chaotic history? (*Things to consider: Separation and/or divorce in the family of origin, numerous changes in residence while growing up, parental psychopathology, a history of physical or sexual abuse.*)

Risk Factors

Suicide does not occur in isolation—compared to matched controls in the general population, people who attempt suicide have been found to have 4 times as many stressful life events in the 6 months leading up to their attempt (Paykel, Prusoff, & Myers, 1975). It is important to consider acute stressors. Life events that have been associated with suicide include interpersonal losses, interpersonal conflict, legal difficulties, and the recent experience of physical and/or emotional abuse (Brent et al., 1993; Marttunen, Aro, & Lönnqvist, 1993).

It is also essential that clinicians be aware of the general "state of mind" that may be indicative of risk. Hopelessness has been associated with risk for suicide. Hopelessness can be conceptualized as a general belief that one's lot in life is unchanging and that one exhibits little control over outcomes in one's life. Clients who express such beliefs should be considered at risk.

Also of importance is whether or not, at the time of the assessment, the person meets criteria for a specific psychiatric diagnosis. About 90% of people who do commit suicide suffer from a major mental disorder (see Kleespies, Deleppo, Gallagher, & Niles, 1999). Three particular Axis I disorders are associated with the highest risk for completed suicide: depression (50% of cases), alcohol and drug abuse (20–25% of cases) and schizophrenia (10% of cases). Clinicians should, of course, be aware that other Axis I disorders are also associated with elevated risk (e.g., posttraumatic stress disorder, eating disorders), as are Axis II disorders, most notably borderline personality disorder and antisocial personality disorder (Duberstein & Conwell, 1997). Both personality disorders are strongly associated with impulsivity, considered to be a risk factor for suicidality. Duberstein and Conwell (1997) have suggested that Axis II disorders may not be independent risk factors for suicide, but rather that the comorbidity of Axis II disorders with Axis I disorders may heighten risk. Of course, suicide risk may also be elevated in persons who do not meet criteria for a psychiatric disorder. However, we should be particularly aware of risk in this population.

According to Joiner et al. (1999), "the most important domain for risk assessment is previous history of suicide attempt" (p. 447). Simply put, people who have attempted suicide in the past are at increased risk for attempting again. Yet it is crucial to keep in mind that between 60 and 70% of people who complete suicide do so on their first attempt (Maris, 1992). In other words, knowing that a person has not attempted in the past should not be interpreted as a protective factor against future attempts.

Another crucial point of assessment is to learn about the nature of the current suicidal symptoms. Joiner, Rudd, and Rajab (1997) found that resolved plans and preparation were major factors in suicidal ideation. During an assessment, it is important to ask the client if he or she has a plan and to assess the lethality of that plan. Is the plan very specific, detailed, and well planned? Does the individual have the means to carry it out (e.g., if he or she plans to commit suicide with a gun, is access to one available to the client?). Also of import is whether the person seems to have the "courage" to carry out the plan.

In Joiner et al.'s (1997) study, the other important factor in suicidal ideation (albeit to a lesser degree than plans and preparation) was suicidal desire. Suicidal desire refers to the degree to which a client desires to die or has difficulty providing reasons for living. Although suicidal desire alone may not constitute extreme risk, the combination of desire and plans/preparation does.

Protective Factors

It is useful to screen for protective factors as well. Therapeutically, questions that tap into this issue may make clients aware that there are some positive aspects of their lives. Furthermore, knowing that clients possess some of these protective factors may help a clinician decide on appropriate interventions (e.g., outpatient as opposed to inpatient care). What are the protective factors against suicide? An important protective factor is social support. We should be more comfortable sending a person with suicidal ideation home with a caring parent or significant other than if the person were going home to an empty house. Heikkinen, Isometsae, Marttunen, Aro, and Lönnqvist (1995) found that people who completed suicide were more likely than people in the general population to live alone and to be either single (never married), divorced, or widowed. Having children under the age of 18 has also been found to be a protective factor. The general idea here is that people who feel that they are depended on by others may be less likely to attempt suicide. We have even known clients who have stated that they would not commit suicide because of a pet that they felt depended on them. Certain personality factors can also serve as protection against suicide. In contrast to impulsivity, which puts people at risk for suicide, people who seem to have good self-control and good problem-solving skills may be at lower risk.

Then What?

By the end of the assessment, you will have two basic paths to take. One is to hospitalize the client. The other is to send the client home with a formalized plan in place for keeping him or her safe, and following up with the person. Most of the time, by the end of a thorough assessment, this decision is not particularly difficult to make. However, if you (and your supervisor) are feeling very unsure, it is best to err on the side of caution. On the one hand, you might have to deal with the client's anger about having been sent to the hospital. On the other hand, the client will still be alive. Dealing with the anger will undoubtedly be easier than dealing with the suicide.

If you believe that the client is not at imminent risk, there are several things to do before you are ready to send the client home. First, you should establish a safety contract with the client. This contract should spell out what the client will do if he or she is feeling suicidal, whether it be going to the emergency room, contacting you or a loved one, or calling a suicide hotline. Clients must be given needed information to follow through with the contract. Specifically, give them the telephone numbers for crisis lines and emergency psychiatric services and let them know how they can reach you. It is also advisable to set an appointment for a telephone contact or for a subsequent session. This can be built into the contract—essentially having the client promise that he or she will "hang on" until you next see each other. These contracts give some structure to clients' lives at a chaotic, confusing time. They also are an important part of recordkeeping, documenting that clients have been given the information they need and that safety nets for them have been put in place.

In addition to contracting for safety, clinicians can do other things to protect their suicidal clients. If the client has the means to actually commit suicide (e.g., a stockpile of pills, a gun), you should help the client plan to dispose of these items. It can also be beneficial to get clients to sign releases so that you can speak to significant others if they find the task too difficult. Supportive friends and family members can be asked to stay with the client, help them rid the house of dangerous objects, and help them get to their next session. It may be necessary to increase the frequency of sessions (e.g., daily, twice a week) with suicidal clients until a reduction in suicidal ideation has been observed.

CLINICIAN-RELATED ROADBLOCKS THAT CAN INTERFERE WITH TREATMENT

Up to this point, we have discussed clinical challenges that arise with the client. Given that therapy is an interpersonal relationship between client and clinician, it is important to also be mindful of what the clinician brings to the table and how our own behavior impacts the therapy. In the next section, we discuss some of these factors and offer suggestions on how to deal with them effectively.

When Clinicians' Own Issues Affect Their Approach to Understanding and Treating a Case

There are bumps along the road of life for all people—even clinicians. An "advantage" of this is that clinicians can draw on their own experiences to better empathize with clients. However, it can be difficult when clinicians have unresolved issues that interfere with their work with clients. For example, clinicians who have issues with shape and weight might have a difficult time "selling" the importance of normalizing eating habits to their clients. Clinicians who have experienced traumas in their lives might begin to have intrusive thoughts and images when working with clients who had similar traumas. Clinicians who have difficulties with mood regulation might find that spending the day talking to depressed clients is just too taxing when they themselves are in the throes of depression. These sorts of reactions can most definitely interfere with the competent delivery of psychotherapy. Difficulties working with certain clients can also arise for clinicians who do not have any significant personal problems. For example, it can be very difficult to listen to very sad or traumatic stories even if you have never experienced a trauma yourself.

Clinicians who have significant psychological difficulties of their own should seek treatment. This is particularly the case when the clinicians' own difficulties interfere in their work with clients or when working with clients exacerbates clinicians' problems. Initially, it can be helpful to discuss these issues in a very general way with your supervisor. However, it is essential that the supervisor not take on the role of clinician. Rather, clinicians with their own problems should seek treatment from an individual who is in no way involved with their training or day-to-day work (as specified in APA code 7.05b). For more minor difficulties, clinicians can actually work through problems on their own before treating clients. For example, if you are assigned a client with a specific phobia of spiders and you are not keen on spiders yourself, it would be best to work on this on your own before treating the client. By doing this, you can then demonstrate exposure exercises (e.g., touching a spider or holding a spider in your hand) in a confident way. In certain situations, it can even be helpful to let the clients know that you also used to fear spiders, but that the kind of treatment you will be doing with them helped you to get past it. While in general we discourage excessive self-disclosure during therapy, sharing a brief example of how a CBT technique helped you through something difficult can be very encouraging for clients.

Clinician Difficulties in the Therapeutic Relationship

It is embarrassing for clinicians to admit that, from time to time, they dislike a client with whom they are working. They might find themselves dreading sessions, and once in session they might have difficulty holding back from saying what they really think of this person sitting across from them. In our "real lives," we would simply choose not to associate with someone whom we dislike, but these reactions are more difficult to handle in the context of the therapeutic relationship.

Before offering a few tips on coping with this situation, it is important to consider what clinicians should do if they frequently, or even always, find that they feel irritated by their clients, are uninterested in them, and have difficulties feeling sympathy for them. If these reactions seem more the norm than the exception, it is best to solicit some guidance from a supervisor. Individuals who habitually experience this type of reaction might not be well suited to a career as a clinician. If such individuals are interested in the field of mental health, there are many other career paths that they can pursue that involve fewer interactions with clients, including administrative positions and positions that are more research oriented. The bottom line is that constant irritation with clients is not good for anyone.

With that being said, let us return to ways of coping with occasional negative reactions to particular clients. First, remind yourself that therapy is time-limited—you will not be seeing this person forever. Although it sounds silly, simply reminding yourself of this fact can be helpful. We have all had the experience of using this tactic and then finding by the end of therapy that some things about the client were actually endearing. Another helpful tip is to remember that you are in control of the tone in therapy and can try to limit factors that you find difficult to handle. For example, a colleague treated a young adult who presented for treatment of a specific disorder. The characteristics of the client that were problematic for the clinician were unrelated to this disorder. The client was terribly racist and was actually a member of a neo-Nazi group. Not surprisingly, the clinician found these views quite troubling. However, the client had not presented for help with changing his views and seemed happy with this aspect of his life. At times during the first few sessions of treatment, the client brought up these views and described to the clinician some of his "extracurricular" activities. The clinician, after consulting with some colleagues on how to deal with this difficult matter, told the client that she felt that these discussions diverted attention from the issues that were supposed to be the focus of treatment. She was honest with the client, telling him that she had difficulties with his views and that although her role was not to change them, she believed treatment would proceed most efficiently if they were not discussed. The client was agreeable to this plan and did very well with the treatment program. Setting ground rules made it easier for the clinician to focus on the client and provide him with the help that he needed. On rare occasions, however, the therapeutic relationship can be so strained that continuing to treat a client would be countertherapeutic. For example, if the aforementioned client did not follow the ground rules and continued to bring up his views or said offensive things to the clinician or other clinic staff, it would certainly have been appropriate to terminate the therapy and refer the client elsewhere.

A final tip is to remember that your reactions to clients are likely very similar to the reactions of people in their "real lives." Use your own reactions as information that can be contributed to the case conceptualization and, in turn, as an indicator for what needs to be worked on in therapy. For example, a colleague was working with a client who constantly interrupted him every time he started to speak. The clinician found this so irritating that he came to dread his sessions with the client. As in the preceding example, the client had presented for treatment of a specific disorder, not for help with interpersonal skills. Nevertheless, the clinician felt that he could not continue with the therapy (or, at the very least, not continue in a good mood) if this issue were not corrected. The clinician finally decided to be direct with the client, point out his ongoing habit of interrupting, and share with the client his reactions to this behavior. Specifically, the clinician said: "When I start to speak, you tend to interrupt. I feel like I never quite finish a sentence. This makes it feel quite difficult to help you. I think our work together would progress better if you heard me out on the suggestions that I make." Not surprisingly, the client told the clinician that other people had given him this same feedback. He found it difficult, however, to break the habit. This admission led the clinician and client to problem solve and devise a plan to work on this issue in the context of their therapy.

In sum, clients sometimes exhibit behaviors or voice beliefs that we find unappealing. In some cases, it is appropriate for clinicians to set limits on clients' behavior, and, in extreme cases, it can even be appropriate to terminate the therapeutic relationship and refer the client elsewhere. In most other cases, clinicians should use their reaction to clients as a window into the client's social world. Clinicians can effectively use their own reactions to help clients improve their social behavior, teaching them specific strategies that might be of great benefit in their lives outside of therapy.

DIFFICULT INTERPERSONAL SITUATIONS IN THE THERAPEUTIC RELATIONSHIP

In the remainder of this chapter we discuss how to deal with difficult interpersonal issues that typically arise early on in the therapeutic relationship. These are issues that come up frequently, but beginning clinicians are rarely taught about how to deal with them. Some advance thought about them makes them much easier to handle.

"My Client Asks Me a Lot of Personal Questions"

The therapeutic relationship is, on a personal level, very one-sided. By the end of even one session with a client, you will have gained all sorts of knowledge about who he or she is—a lot of it very personal in nature. In contrast, even after working together for many months, the client knows very little about the clinician. Some clients do not seem to mind this and rarely ask questions of a personal nature. Others appear more curious, asking your age, where you live, where you come from, or whether you are in a relationship. Clinicians of different orientations have different views on personal questions, with some schools seeing them infused with meaning and some ascribing less weight. In our opinion, it seems appropriate to handle questions (and what they might mean) on a case-by-case basis.

Being Asked about Age and Experience

Being asked about age and level of experience can be particularly trying for beginning clinicians. Particularly if you look younger than you are, these questions/statements may come up quite regularly—and for some time after you are no longer a beginning clinician! One of us continues to get asked this question regularly and (for better or worse) has given a great deal of thought to how to respond. It is our sense that when clients ask about the age of their clinicians, they are actually interested in the clinician's level of experience, both in therapy and in life (e.g., a couple with marital problems might wonder how a young, unmarried clinician could relate to their problems, and thus help them effectively). Therefore, a good way to deal with the question is to respond according to level of experience, not your actual chronological age. For example, if a client says, "You look very young," you can respond by saying "I have just started my third year of the doctoral program here" or "I've been on the faculty here for 3 years now." Similarly, if a client with marital problems says "If you're not married, I don't see how you could help," you can respond with "I've worked well with a number of couples and I hope I can be of help to you as well."

When clients are concerned about the clinician's level of experience, they will sometimes ask about it directly. As a beginning clinician, it might very well be true that you have never seen a client with concerns like the client asking the question—in fact, you might never have seen a client at all! Although we do not want to lie to our clients, we also do not want to emphasize our lack of experience. In these situations, a good strategy is to emphasize the expertise of the place at which you work and the individuals who are supervising you. If a client asks, "Have you seen any clients who have panic disorder like I do?" you might respond, "This center is a world-renowned treatment and research center for people with panic disorder. The treatment offered here is really cutting-edge and I receive excellent supervision." By focusing on your training setting, rather than on yourself (the inexperienced clinician), you can respond to this type of question in a positive but truthful way.

What should you do if these tactics do not work, and a client continues to voice concerns about working with a beginning clinician? One option is to return to the stance of a scientist—"I understand your hesitancy here. Why don't we get started and see in a few sessions how you feel that things are going?" This stance is particularly effective when clients have few other options. Trying therapy with an inexperienced clinician is typically considered a better choice than doing nothing at all. In our experience, few clients continue to complain about being paired with an inexperienced clinician once they begin to see some benefit from the therapy.

Continuing difficulties with a beginning clinician can also inform the case conceptualization. We treated a client who was very concerned about having a young, novice clinician. She was unhappy with the arrangement but could not afford treatment with someone with more experience. For the first few sessions, the client continually brought up the issue—"You wouldn't understand that since you've never treated someone with problems like mine" or "I bet you don't know what to do with someone as severe as me." The clinician sought supervision about this problem—she did not want to spend every session trying to convince the client of her abilities. Her supervisor advised her to confront the client directly about her discomfort. This turned out to be excellent advice. The client explained that she would not have a significant problem with an inexperienced clinician who was 40—but having one who was in her mid-20s was terrible. The client, also in her mid-20s, was significantly impaired. She was not in school, was working at a menial job, and had just left a relationship because of her psychological problems. Looking across the room at a person of the same age who was progressing successfully with her education and career (and presumably had a fulfilling life outside of these arenas as well) was "a slap in the face" for this client.

Her clinician reacted to this explanation with empathy and told the client that she was sorry that this was so difficult for her. She then asked if there was any way that they could put these thoughts to good use in the therapy. The client explained that her reactions to the clinician made her realize how much she wanted to have the life of someone in their 20s, rather than the isolated life she was leading right now, where she was not meeting her potential. After this session, the issue of the clinician's inexperience never came up again.

Obviously, all cases do not end so positively. Some clients steadfastly refuse to work with an inexperienced clinician. In these cases, time should not be spent trying to reason with clients or convince them that they are wrong. Rather, an appropriate referral should be provided to the client.

Other Personal Questions

A personal question that often comes up early in the therapeutic relationship is whether the clinician has any personal experience with the difficulties that the client is having. Some people do naturally gravitate toward areas that have personal resonance for them, and, in some settings, sharing personal experience is acceptable. However, this is the exception and not the rule. By sharing with a client your own experiences, you are taking the focus off the client, and this is not therapeutically beneficial.

The real issue underlying this kind of question is that clients want to feel understood and confident that you will be able to identify with their concerns. With this in mind, the question can be answered in a few different ways. First, you can refer again to your therapy experience—"I've worked with a lot of clients who have panic disorder. That has really helped me to understand the experience of having panic attacks and how it feels to fear a lot of situations because of them." Furthermore, you can try to normalize clients' difficulties and point out that on some level, you have had similar experiences—"Social anxiety is very common. Just like most people, I get anxious sometimes in social situations. So, yes, I can understand some of the feelings you've been telling me about today." Both of these strategies help the client to feel understood, without the clinician revealing much personal information.

A whole host of other personal questions can come up in the therapeutic relationship. Many personal questions are completely innocuous, and answering them should not feel uncomfortable. A client might ask where you are from, particularly if you speak with an accent or if they look at your diplomas on the wall and see that you were not educated in the city in which you are currently living and practicing. Before holidays or vacations, clients might ask you about your plans. It seems more damaging to the therapeutic relationship to explain why you cannot answer questions like these than to simply say, "I am from Canada" or "I am going to see my family for the holidays."

Other questions are not quite as easy to handle, particularly those of a very personal nature (e.g., your relationship status, where you live, exactly where you are going to be on your holidays, etc.). It can be difficult to deal with these questions, and for clients who persistently ask personal questions, it is worth addressing this issue directly. It can be helpful to acknowledge the differential that is inherent in the therapeutic relationship—the client bares all and the clinician is a relatively blank slate. Once you have acknowledged to clients that you realize that this is difficult, it is important to explain why this is the case—that therapy is about them and helping them with their difficulties and that anything which takes the focus away from this goal is detrimental.

As we have already noted, it is important to identify the function of various client behaviors. A client who repeatedly tries to turn the focus onto the clinician might be trying to delay discussing his or her own issues. This hypothesis can be presented to the client and discussed. Clients who try to get chummy with the clinician might be lonely and lacking meaningful relationships in their own lives. Again, this can be good fodder for therapy in that clients can be encouraged to start applying some of their interpersonal skills (e.g., asking personal questions in a socially appropriate way) to new relationships outside of therapy.

"What Do I Do When a Client Brings Me a Gift?"

We all love to receive gifts from friends and family members. However, our feelings about gifts can be quite different when the "givers" are our clients. You might work in a setting where accepting gifts from clients is completely forbidden. Most settings, however, will not have a clearly stated policy and you will have to work out how to deal with the issue as it comes up.

Gifts offered during therapy are a bit trickier to deal with than a single gift offered at the end of a successful course of therapy. Similarly, gifts offered outside the context of some formal gift-giving occasion (e.g., Christmas) likely have a more complex meaning. It seems to be a generally accepted rule that gifts of high monetary value should never be accepted from clients. Similarly, never accept cash gifts ("tips") from clients. Caution should also be taken if clients give gifts to you of minimal value, but on a frequent basis. Although such situations do not come up frequently, you should become comfortable with turning these kinds of gifts down. You can explain to clients that accepting expensive gifts or gifts of money is against the policy of your place of work. If clients are insistent or attempt to give you gifts repeatedly, you should explore the issue with them and consider how this behavior might influence your understanding of the case. Clients may give gifts to clinicians as a means of ingratiation. For example, they may think that if they are generous with you, you will agree to see them more frequently. Other clients may worry about whether or not you like them and may hope that, by giving gifts, you will like them more. Clearly, these motives behind gift giving are problematic and should be dealt with through the use of cognitive techniques. As with so many other issues we have been discussing, client behavior in session likely mirrors their behavior outside of session. Believing that one can use gifts to "buy friends and influence people" is not appropriate, and correcting such beliefs in session can be very helpful to clients' lives outside of session.

The aforementioned situations (bringing gifts to almost every session, giving very expensive gifts) are obviously problematic. Yet, it can also be difficult to know how to react to gifts that are given at holiday times or at the end of treatment. As noted earlier, some settings might have very clear "no gift" policies; in settings that do not, the cardinal rule of not accepting very expensive gifts or gifts of money should be followed. Accepting gifts of lesser value, particularly at the last session of treatment, can be fine and, in fact, refusing these gifts can offend clients who truly want to thank you for your help. As in the case of answering personal questions about yourself, the decision to accept or return gifts should be made on a case-by-case basis. In some cases, accepting gifts will not "feel right." Trust your gut instincts, acknowledge the client's generosity, and clearly explain why you cannot accept the gift.

"My Client Invited Me to a Social Event"

As difficult as it is to gracefully deal with receiving gifts from clients, an even more awkward situation is being invited to a social event by a client. The general rule of thumb is that we should never participate in social activities like playing golf or going for coffee outside of therapy with our clients. If clients repeatedly ask you to do so, it is worth considering how it might influence the case conceptualization and how it can be addressed in therapy. Typically, these frequent invitations are a sign of loneliness or misplaced attraction, and time is much better spent helping the client to establish appropriate social relationships outside of the context of therapy.

An interesting question to pose is whether there are ever exceptions to the rule of not participating in social events with clients. We recently encountered an interesting situation that helped us to think more clearly about this issue. One of our colleagues was invited to a religious event for one of her pediatric clients. The clinician had worked with this child for quite some time and had become close with the entire family as they went through some particularly trying events. The child felt very strongly about having her clinician present at this important occasion.

The clinician brought the dilemma to a group supervision meeting. After much weighing of the pros and cons, it was decided that the child would be very disappointed and hurt if the clinician did not attend. The clinician set up a meeting with the family to discuss what she would say at the event if other guests asked how she knew the family. The child, being very astute, had already thought this dilemma though and had come up with an explanation with which she felt comfortable. Once all these parameters were worked out, the clinician and her colleagues felt reasonably comfortable with the plan.

It was interesting to hear about the outcome of the event. The child was absolutely thrilled to have her clinician present. She said it was one of the best parts of her special day. The clinician, however, found the experience very stressful! She used the explanation that she and the family had come up with when people asked her how she came to be at the event. Yet, all the while, she felt uncomfortable doing so and felt on edge throughout, fearing that she would slip in some way and break confidentiality. Given the same scenario again, this clinician said that she would decline the invitation.

How then does one go about declining an invitation without insulting the client? The best way to do this is to first express great gratitude for the invitation. Then, explain to clients why you make it a rule to not attend such events. The major reason, of course, is to protect the privacy of clients. If clients have difficulty with this explanation, it can be useful to further explore why it is so important to them that you do attend. As in the case of social invitations (e.g., to get coffee or go to a movie), it might be that clients are lonely and consider their clinician to be one of their closest "friends." Again, this can be used to motivate clients to work on establishing social ties in their lives outside of therapy.

An added complication is what to do about gifts if you are invited to events like weddings, religious ceremonies (e.g., first communions, Bar Mitzvahs), or graduations. Even if you do not attend the event, you should acknowledge the invitation in some way besides simply telling the client that you appreciated it. This is an issue that the clinician just described had to deal with. During group supervision, her colleagues suggested a donation to a charity. The clinician made a donation to the locale humane society in the child's honor, since she was very passionate about animals. Some clinicians might feel more comfortable just sending a card.

"My Client Seems to Be Flirting with Me"

A situation that most clinicians dread is the experience of a client flirting with them. "Flirtation" can take many guises. Some clients will compliment their clinicians on their appearance or manner of dress. Some will be quite overt about their interest, such as saying "I'd love to date a woman like you" or even asking the clinician out on a date. Even more difficult are more subtle cues, such as a client looking at you in an inappropriate manner.

When clients engage in overtly inappropriate behavior, keep in mind that you can set limits in the session—"I don't think it's appropriate for you to keep asking me out on dates," for example. It is more useful, however, to try to figure out why clients are behaving in this way toward you. How does it fit into the case conceptualization and how can you address the problem productively in therapy? Generally, clients who behave in this way are having difficulties with romantic relationships in their lives outside therapy. They might have very limited social interactions—in fact, they might spend more time (and more time speaking about personal matters) with you than with anyone else in their lives. Similarly, the kinds of difficulties that clients have might preclude them from establishing meaningful relationships. They might have problems approaching people at all, or they might be fine approaching people but then behave in such a way that others do not want to establish relationships with them. Your interactions with clients will most likely shed light on the nature of their interpersonal difficulties. You can then use your own insights as a means of helping clients work on these problems during therapy.

Clearly, if clients behave so inappropriately that you feel uncomfortable in the room with them or feel as if you are unable to provide them with good treatment, therapy should be discontinued and appropriate referrals made. In such situations, ongoing consultation with your supervisor is essential, and the decision to terminate therapy should be made with his or her support.

Chapter 8

■　■　■

THE NEXT SESSIONS
Teaching the Core Techniques

Now that we know how to conceptualize and manage some of the challenges that can come up in the early stages of treatment, let's return to the process of CBT. In most CBT protocols, the sessions following psychoeducation involve teaching clients the skills that they will use during the remainder of therapy. Typically, new skills are gradually introduced over a few sessions, with the expectation that clients will add these skills to ones acquired in previous sessions.

The content of these early sessions of CBT will vary greatly, depending on the focus of treatment. In CBT for bulimia, for example, early treatment sessions include the prescription of regular eating patterns and learning about self-control strategies that can help clients to decrease the occurrence of binge eating (see Wilson, Fairburn, & Agras, 1997). Slightly later in Wilson et al.'s protocol, clients are also taught more standard CBT techniques, including problem solving and cognitive restructuring. After completing psychoeducation in Barlow's panic control treatment (see Craske & Barlow, 2001), clients are taught breathing control and cognitive restructuring. Later in the protocol, clients commence interoceptive and *in vivo* exposures as a means of confronting their feared physical symptoms, as well as the situations that they fear will bring on symptoms of panic. The best way to learn these techniques is to read the manuals, watch more experienced clinicians do them, and then get feedback from supervisors as you begin to apply them with your own patients. To illustrate just one application of CBT, we will continue with the case of Michael. His treatment plan consisted of two core techniques: cognitive restructuring and graduated exposures.

SESSION 3: INTRODUCING COGNITIVE RESTRUCTURING

In Session 3, Michael's clinician followed the basic session format by first checking in on his week, reviewing his self-monitoring homework, and then setting the session agenda in collaboration with Michael. As proposed in the treatment plan, the main content of the session was to start the process of cognitive restructuring.

Most CBT manuals explain how to do cognitive restructuring, but, in keeping with the case of Michael, we focus on how it is done in the Hope et al. (2000) manual. By now, Michael has been introduced several times to the basic idea that there is a relationship between events, thoughts, and feelings. This idea that our interpretations of events, not the events themselves, cause negative feelings and behaviors is crucial to CBT, and it serves as the rationale for cognitive restructuring. The previous sessions' homework involved Michael monitoring his thoughts, feelings, and behaviors in anxiety-provoking situations. These monitoring sheets—or other concerns brought into the session—can now provide the raw material for the cognitive restructuring process.

To begin to get a flavor of cognitive restructuring, Michael and his therapist focused on one event that had happened during his week: a sermon he had given at a local nursing home. This sermon was the "activating event" that got Michael's social anxiety going. After the sermon, he recorded the following thoughts on his self-monitoring sheet: "I messed that up so badly," "I'm never going to get this right," and "I'm never going to succeed at this." The consequences of thinking this way were that Michael felt very down for the rest of the day (emotional reaction) and when one of his classmates suggested going for a quick dinner together, he declined and ate by himself (behavioral reaction). Identifying the activating event, belief, and consequence (in terms of feelings and behaviors) for this particular situation helped Michael to see that the sermon, in and of itself, did not cause him to feel bad—rather, his interpretation of the situation did. He immediately accepted the idea that our interpretation of events is more problematic than events themselves and started to understand why it might be helpful to reframe negative thoughts.

Michael's therapist then helped him to take a step back to the very beginning of the activating event: What was he thinking about before he even got to the nursing home where he was giving his sermon? These automatic thoughts included:

- "I'm definitely going to mess up."
- "They'll think I'm incompetent."
- "They'll know that I am going to be a total failure as a priest."
- "If I stumble over a word, it will be a disaster."

He was then asked what kind of emotions his automatic thoughts caused him to have. Michael reported that these thoughts made him feel anxious, sad, and angry. He recognized that they put him in a very bad frame of mind for going to do the sermon.

Seeing that Michael was quite adept at identifying automatic thoughts and recognizing their connection to his emotions, his therapist started to teach him about various kinds of thinking errors, outlined in the Hope et al. (2000) manual beginning on page 84. There are many labels available to describe the logical errors inherent in automatic thoughts. Being able, first, to identify and, second, to label automatic thoughts are the initial steps in cognitive restructuring. In effect, by labeling a thought we recognize what is "wrong" with it. One thing to be mindful of is that labeling thoughts as dysfunctional can cause some clients to feel as if something is wrong with them. It is important to communicate to clients that everyone has negative automatic thoughts, and the problem with them is that they get in the way of people doing what they want to do. In doing cognitive restructuring, the *person* is not labeled as dysfunctional, the *thought* is.

With that caveat in mind, let's consider what to do with an automatic thought once it is identified. It can be very dull to hear a clinician run through a laundry list of possible thinking errors. Instead, it is best to use the clients' own experiences and thoughts, together with Socratic questioning, to help clients begin to see the thinking errors for themselves. For Michael, "I'm definitely going to mess up" and "I'm going to be a total failure as a priest" were both examples of fortune-telling errors—he predicted that he would fail at his speech and at his career as a priest in general before having embarked on either. "They'll think I'm incompetent" was an example of a mind-reading error—assuming we can read the minds of others and know what they think of us. Michael's belief about stumbling over a word was used to demonstrate the concept of mental filter—focusing on one negative aspect of an experience while ignoring the sum total of an experience. Michael's clinician also pointed out to him that he had done a fair bit of "labeling"—using negative labels for himself like "incompetent" and "total failure"—which he likely would not use to describe other people.

Once Michael became adept at describing different kinds of negative thoughts, his clinician introduced the idea of "arguing back," or disputing his negative thoughts. A goal of cognitive restructuring is to help clients become their own "devil's advocate," questioning the validity of their thoughts and examining whether they are helpful or harmful. To accomplish this goal, Michael was provided with a list of possible questions that he could use to dispute automatic thoughts. These were also taken from the Hope et al. (2000) manual. The use of some of these "disputing questions" is illustrated in the following dialogue:

CLINICIAN: So, let's start with the thought, "I'm definitely going to mess up." What question could you ask yourself to challenge this thought?

MICHAEL: Well, I could ask myself, "Do I have any evidence that I will mess up or that I will be a total failure as a priest?"

CLINICIAN: Excellent. Now, there is also an important next step in the process.

MICHAEL: What's that?

CLINICIAN: The next step is to respond to your question. Do you have any evidence for these beliefs? Let's start with the belief about messing up the sermon.

MICHAEL: Well, as we already kind of talked about, I hadn't done the sermon yet when I thought these things. So, how could I know?

CLINICIAN: Right. Any other evidence you can draw on?

MICHAEL: This isn't the first sermon I've done. Is that what you're referring to?

CLINICIAN: I don't know. Why don't you follow through with that thought?

MICHAEL: I've never totally screwed up in other sermons.

CLINICIAN: What's generally happened?

MICHAEL: I generally do okay. I worry so much beforehand and then it turns out fine. But, for some reason, when giving a sermon comes up again, the fear is still there.

CLINICIAN: Okay. That's useful to know. We'll give that some thought as we proceed with the treatment. How about the thought, "They'll think I'm incompetent."

MICHAEL: Well, first of all, we already discussed how I can't read people's minds. I understand that. But after sermons I still feel that the parishioners thought I was incompetent. I think that thought is worse than the one I have before doing the sermon.

CLINICIAN: So, what can you do about that thought?

MICHAEL: I have no idea.

CLINICIAN: Let's look at our sheet of disputes. Any thoughts?

MICHAEL: I could ask myself, "Do I know for certain that they thought I was incompetent?"

CLINICIAN: What would the answer be?

MICHAEL: I can't know what people are thinking.

CLINICIAN: Let's consider a few more questions here. What does it mean to be incompetent?

MICHAEL: Oh, you know, a person who stumbles over all their words and doesn't make any sense. Just kind of a jumble of stuff with no coherence.

CLINICIAN: Would you notice anything from other people if you were to speak in that way?

MICHAEL: Well, people would probably look confused.

CLINICIAN: Is that something you notice when you speak? Do you have evidence to suggest that people are confused?

MICHAEL: No. If I really think about, I actually have some evidence that would go against that.

CLINICIAN: Really? Tell me about that.

MICHAEL: After my sermons, people come up to me to chat about them. Actually, some parishioners write e-mails to me as well, wanting to discuss some topic further.

CLINICIAN: So?

MICHAEL: So, if they were confused, they probably couldn't do this.

CLINICIAN: Michael, that's a great observation to make. Often, socially anxious people are so focused on picking up support for their negative beliefs that they miss out on information that runs counter to them.

MICHAEL: Yeah. I had never thought about that.

CLINICIAN: Okay, one more question before we move on. We can't guarantee that people's feared outcomes will never occur. You have a lot of evidence for making sermons without "messing up." All of us, from time to time, make a speech of some sort and feel less than happy with it. Maybe we didn't get enough sleep the night before and couldn't concentrate well or maybe something very stressful was going on in our lives and we just couldn't get focused. The likelihood of having a real disaster is quite small, but let's consider what would happen if you did stumble over a lot of words and delivered a sermon that was not particularly coherent.

MICHAEL: Gosh, that would be terrible.

CLINICIAN: Well, let's really think about it. What would be so bad about this situation?

MICHAEL: I'd be embarrassed.

CLINICIAN: Okay. And what's so bad about that?

MICHAEL: Well, it *feels* terrible.

CLINICIAN: Yes, it can feel pretty bad. Would there be any other consequence?

MICHAEL: I might lose my job.

CLINICIAN: Really? After one botched sermon?

MICHAEL: I don't know. I guess it could happen.

CLINICIAN: Gee, if that were the case, I would have lost my job a while ago! I've messed up a couple of lectures and talks here and there.

MICHAEL: I guess you're right. You're saying that I'd have to really mess up a bunch right in a row to start seeing any consequences.

CLINICIAN: That's what I think. What do you think?

MICHAEL: I agree. I guess really all I'm left with is feeling embarrassed. Maybe feeling more nervous for the sermon that comes after the botched one.

CLINICIAN: What do you make of that?

MICHAEL: Well, it sounds like less of a big deal than I always make it out to be.

CLINICIAN: Hmmm. Pretty good take-home message, isn't it?

MICHAEL: Yeah. It sure is. Kind of makes me wonder what I've been freaking out about all these years.

CLINICIAN: Sounds like things could be a bit easier from here on in.

MICHAEL: Absolutely.

Michael's clinician led him through the disputing process with a few more automatic thoughts and then, as per the treatment protocol, introduced to Michael the concept of a rational response. A rational response is a short summary statement of what was learned during cognitive restructuring that a client can use to stay focused and rational in situations that provoke social anxiety. After this concept was explained to Michael, his clinician helped him to develop one to use for his next sermon. Michael came up with the rational response "I can't know the outcome until I do the task."

Following this initial session of cognitive work, Michael was asked to monitor his automatic thoughts during the week and work through the process of disputing them on his own. He was asked to do this in writing and to bring his homework with him to the next session. Michael was reminded that the homework did not have to be perfect; it was simply important to start seeing how cognitive restructuring worked and to have some material to bring in to the next session. At the close of the session, Michael came up with the following "take-home message" to add to his list: "I don't have to take my thoughts as laws. I should question them and see if they are rational."

SESSION 4: CONTINUING COGNITIVE RESTRUCTURING
AND PLANNING THE FIRST EXPOSURE

As in earlier sessions, Session 4 started with a check-in about Michael's week and a review of his homework—in this case, cognitive restructuring records. Michael seemed rather ebullient when he arrived for this session. He had really embraced cognitive restructuring and had found that he was slightly less anxious about some of the situations that came up during the week. For example, the evening before the session, Michael was preparing for a class he had that morning, in which each student was always called on at least once during every class. Typically, Michael would stay up most of the night before this particular class, making sure he knew all the material perfectly since he knew he would be called on but did not know what he would be asked. At about 11 P.M., he was getting tired and really wished he could just go to sleep. This thought was countered by another thought: "If I don't spend some more time on this, I'm going to make a total fool of myself." When Michael realized that he had just had an automatic thought, he pulled out his homework sheets and worked through the process of cognitive restructuring. He came to two major realizations: (1) He had no evidence that he would make a total fool of himself, and (2) he was usually so tired in class that he was not at his best. He came up with the rational response: "A fresh mind might do me good." With that, he went to sleep. In class that morning, he knew the answer to the question he was asked and even felt good about his response.

This was a pivotal experience for Michael in a number of ways. He took initiative for his treatment, applying what he had learned in therapy in a very practical and useful way. This demonstrated to him that he did have some control over his situation and that it was not certain that he would be paralyzed by social anxiety forever. In addition, Michael essentially designed an exposure for himself—he decided to go to class less prepared than usual and see what would happen. In doing so, Michael experienced a shift in his beliefs. This was partly accomplished through cognitive restructuring, but solidified through an actual experience in which Michael disconfirmed his beliefs. Using Socratic questioning, Michael's clinician made sure that he recognized this progress as clearly as she did.

At this point in the session, Michael and his therapist reviewed his other cognitive restructuring homework from the week. They spent some time "fine-tuning"—his therapist offered pointers for different ways to dispute thoughts and suggested ways to come up with more concise rational responses. It was quite clear, however, that Michael understood cognitive restructuring, and he had certainly seen a positive impact of it during the prior week.

The first exposure, which was to happen during the next session, was then planned. Michael and his clinician decided that this first exposure would entail having a casual conversation with a person whom he had not yet met. This situation was rated a "50" on the fear and avoidance hierarchy (see Figure 6.2). Moderately anxiety-provoking situations are typically considered good choices for the initial exposure. They agreed that the first exposure would occur with a male confederate, since a casual conversation with a woman was further up Michael's hierarchy. Getting this plan in place allowed time for the clinician to locate a confederate to participate in the exposure.

SESSION 5: DOING THE FIRST EXPOSURE

In Session 5, Michael and his clinician checked in, set an agenda, and reviewed his homework, which again was to work through the process of cognitive restructuring as anxiety-provoking situations came up in his life. Michael had again done a good job of completing the homework and had a few more opportunities during the week to use cognitive restructuring to help him cope with stressful situations. Of note, Michael was also doing his homework "less perfectly." He was no longer typing it, was using point form rather than beautifully constructed sentences, and seemed less concerned about spelling mistakes than he had been at the beginning of treatment.

Before getting started with the first exposure, Michael and his therapist reviewed the purpose of exposures: to see that anxiety will naturally diminish even in very anxiety-provoking situations and to have the opportunity to test out his beliefs. The parameters of the exposure were then defined. Michael and his clinician agreed that he would have a conversation with a male stranger, sitting down in chairs, with no set topic to discuss. In the case of Michael, a graduate student who worked in the clinic where he was being treated served as the "confederate" for the exposure. This individual was simply told to act like himself and have a conversation with Michael as he would with a fellow classmate or someone he met at a party. Any person in a clinic setting can play this role—a receptionist, another clinician, the business manager. Some clinics, however, do not have access to such people and in these cases, the exposure can be carried out with the clinician.

With the parameters for the exposure set, Michael was asked to identify his automatic thoughts, dispute them, and come up with a rational response to take with him into the exposure. Michael's automatic thoughts mostly centered around not knowing what to say during the conversation, resulting in awkward silences. After disputing these thoughts, Michael came up with the rational response, "Conversation is a two-way street," to remind himself that the other individual also had some responsibility for carrying on the conversation. Before beginning the exposure, Michael was asked to set some goals. Initially, Michael selected the goal "Not being anxious." Michael's clinician encouraged him to instead select an observable, measurable goal based on what he *did* in the situation, rather than on how he *felt*. Michael set the goal of telling the other person three things about himself and also asking the other person three questions in return.

Michael followed through with the planned exposure. The conversation went well, with Michael sharing information about himself and also asking questions of the confederate to learn more about him. The session did not end with the conclusion of the conversation, however. Although an exposure activity might seem like it went extremely well to the clinician, it is possible that the client came away with quite a different impression. Therefore, the final step of the exposure technique is to engage in postprocessing and to discuss with the client what he learned from the experience.

First, Michael was asked if he achieved his goal. He recognized that he had, in fact, shared a number of things about himself and had also learned a lot about the confederate by asking questions in return. Michael's clinician asked if he had been anxious during the conversation and he replied that he had, particularly at the beginning. His clinician then emphasized that the conversation went well and that Michael achieved his goals despite feeling anxious. Next, Michael was asked to reevaluate his initial automatic thoughts. Michael reported that they had little validity—he did have things to say, there were no long gaps in the conversations, and the conversation flowed very well. Finally, Michael was asked what he learned from the experience. He explained that the best learning tool was to always distinguish between feelings and behaviors. He liked the idea that what mattered in social situations was what he did, not how he felt. With further discussion about this, Michael was able to recognize that he often left social situations judging them on feelings (e.g., "The sermon was a disaster because I *felt* so anxious") and that this type of judgment influenced his beliefs in the subsequent times he had to enter that same situation (e.g., "I was nervous last time, so this time is going to be a disaster too").

With the first in-session exposure complete, Michael was assigned a similar exposure for homework. A few of his classmates had invited him to have lunch with him the next day. He would typically avoid doing so for the same reasons he expressed prior to doing the exposure—he worried that he would not have anything to say. For homework, he was asked to accept the lunch invitation and to treat it as an exposure. His clinician recommended that he look back at his list of "take-home messages" if he hesitated about going. Following this first in-session exposure, Michael had added two take-home messages that would likely be helpful: "Doing it was much easier than thinking about it," and "It is important to judge events on what you did, not on how you felt."

Michael was also given a handout to help guide him through the exposure, which included preparation before it (cognitive restructuring, coming up with a rational response, stating some goals) and debriefing after it (Did you accomplish your goals? What did you learn? etc.). Since the exposure would be happening the very next day, Michael and his clinician set up a phone session for later that afternoon. This served two purposes. When clients first do exposures, they can be their own worst enemies, falling into their old patterns of judging success based on how they *felt*, not on what they did. A phone check-in would help to ensure that Michael had done a good job of processing the exposure once it was done. Another benefit of a phone check-in is that it provides the opportunity to troubleshoot if a client agrees to do an exposure but then cannot carry through with it once he or she is home. If this had been the case with Michael, his clinician could have given him some tips for completing the assigned homework, or, alternatively, another exposure could have been assigned if the initial one was too difficult or if the opportunity to do it had passed. In this way, the entire week until the next session is not wasted and clients do not spend the whole week feeling demoralized about their inability to carry through with the homework plan.

SESSIONS 6–10: CONTINUING COGNITIVE RESTRUCTURING AND EXPOSURES TO FEARED SITUATIONS

Treatment for Michael continued to run very smoothly for the next five sessions. In session, he had a few more casual conversations with both male and female confederates and delivered a number of sermons with varying levels of preparation. He also completed assigned homework and seized opportunities for additional exposures whenever things naturally came up in his life.

This engagement in the treatment was paralleled by behavioral and cognitive changes. Michael noticed a significant decrease in his anxiety in his day-to-day life and experienced a significant improvement in his functioning. He was doing well in his classes (with far less preparation), taking opportunities to do sermons and interact with parishioners (rather than avoiding them), and had become chummy with a number of his classmates. Over these 10 sessions, he experienced a major shift in his beliefs about making mistakes and being rejected. He came to recognize that he made mistakes with far less frequency than he would have expected, and that when he did so (e.g., stumbling over a word during a sermon or telling a joke during lunch that people did not "get"), there really were no consequences. Parishioners did not stop coming to his sermons if he made a mistake, and his classmates did not stop being his friends if he told a silly joke. If anything, Michael saw very positive consequences of his increasingly social behavior.

How did the case conceptualization and treatment plan shift over this time? First, it became evident that it would not be necessary to spend a full 20 weeks on treatment for social phobia. Michael had made gains very quickly and was seizing every opportunity that came up in his life to work on his social anxiety. Michael's therapist revised the treatment plan to include two or three more exposure sessions and then two sessions to discuss relapse prevention and goal setting.

What about the other items on Michael's problem list? What was their status, and would time need to be allocated to deal with them? As treatment proceeded, it became clear that social anxiety had likely been standing in the way of Michael's being able to confidently make a decision about whether or not to pursue the priesthood. Once social anxiety became less of a concern, Michael started enjoying his work to a much greater degree and could easily picture a life that included interacting with parishioners, leading religious services, doing sermons, and being involved in other aspects of religious life.

As Michael became more confident about his work, he also started to believe that his family was more "on board" with his choices. His parents had come to visit a few times and had attended services he led. They had been impressed with these services and with the way that Michael interacted with the churchgoers at the end of the service. While Michael knew they would still be unhappy if he decided to enter the priesthood since he would be giving up having his own family, he started to accept this. He had some good discussions on the topic with his parents, and he felt that all of them had an opportunity to voice their opinions on the matter. Ultimately, Michael came to see that if he became a priest, his parents would continue to support him and that they would have to handle their disappointment about his not marrying nor having children.

On that topic, Michael's own thoughts about marrying and having children did not come up during these sessions of therapy. His clinician did not push the issue, particularly since it was not an issue Michael came into therapy wanting to discuss. However, as we discuss in Chapter 10, the issue did arise later. At this point, let's shift for the remainder of the chapter to a discussion of how to document our work with clients.

KEEPING GOOD CLIENT RECORDS

The Why of Recordkeeping

Client records are important for two reasons—legal and ethical accountability and good clinical practice. Let us first consider accountability. Keeping good records is an excellent way to protect yourself should you be subject to any disciplinary action. As with psychological reports, you should always be mindful that the chart is not "for your eyes only." Records might eventually be read by other professionals or by clients themselves. At times, records are subpoenaed for legal cases. Keeping all these "possible readers" in mind, clinicians should avoid making derogatory comments about clients. Records should be succinct, legibly written, and should avoid the use of jargon where possible. Most importantly, records should be complete, including an account of all sessions, all contact with clients outside of sessions, and all conversations with other professionals or other people in clients' lives. A good reminder for the therapist to keep in mind is that, as far as accountability is concerned, "If it is not documented, it did not happen."

More relevant on a day-to-day basis is the clinical usefulness of client records. Particularly if you are seeing multiple clients, the record serves as a way for you to refresh your memory about the client before each session. Even when remembering the details of clients' lives is not a problem, the record also helps with session planning—it should contain information about the homework that was assigned and what plans had been made for the upcoming session.

Writing progress notes is also very useful in terms of case conceptualization. By dedicating time after each session to writing a note, you force yourself to reexamine the case and decide whether adjustments need to be made to your understanding of it or to your plan for treatment.

One additional advantage of client records is that they facilitate communication between professionals. This is particularly important with beginning clinicians who might pass cases on to other clinicians before the course of treatment is complete (due to changing practicum sites, graduation, etc.). Being able to read another clinician's notes on the case is an invaluable experience. When discussing cases with other professionals (e.g., psychiatrists, clinicians beginning to treat clients whom you treated in the past, etc.), keep in mind that you may not want to pass along all of your session notes to them. First, doing so is not a very effective means of communication—reading through many sessions' worth of notes can be very time-consuming. Furthermore, notes may include information that the other professional does not need to know in order to do his or her work effectively. Having kept clear records, however, will allow you to put together a summary report that would be a more succinct and relevant document for other professionals to read.

The Content of Records

An overview of typical content in a client record is listed in Table 8.1. Records should first include demographic information—the client's name, date of birth, contact information (address and phone number), and information for an emergency contact. If there are any special instructions for making contact (e.g., do not send mail to home address, do not leave the name of your clinic on phone messages, etc.), these should be noted in the record. You may also want to include contact in-

TABLE 8.1. Overview of Content of Client Records

- Demographic information
   Client name
   Date of birth
   Client contact information
   Special contact instructions
   Whom to contact in an emergency
- Signed consent forms
   Consent to assessment
   Consent to treatment
   Permission to speak with other health care professionals
   Agreement on fees, missed appointments
- Initial assessment report
- Progress (session) notes (signed by supervisor, if necessary)
- Completed self-monitoring forms, hierarchies, homework assignments, other materials
- Record of all contacts with client (e.g., phone calls, e-mails)
- Record of any contact with other individuals involved in the case

formation for other professionals with whom you are planning to communicate about the case.

The record should also include all signed consent forms (consent to assessment, consent to treatment), as well as signed forms providing permission to speak to other health care professionals. A signed agreement on fees, missed appointments, and the like should also be in the client's record, as should the initial assessment report.

The record should additionally include the progress notes that you write after each session with the client. As with assessment reports, there is a lot of variation in progress notes. It is best to ask your supervisors how they prefer progress notes to be written. Over time, you will develop your own style. Wiger (1998) has recommended the DAP format, which stands for data, assessment, and plan. We have created a sample progress note from one of Michael's therapy sessions, which appears as Figure 8.1.

The client's chart should also include other materials, including completed self-monitoring sheets or other homework assignments, hierarchies, thought records, and the like. This "additional material" will obviously vary greatly, depending on the focus of treatment. Clinicians should not be the only ones keeping records of the therapy—clients should also be encouraged to maintain their handouts and forms in a folder or binder. This reinforces the collaborative nature of the therapy. Some clients like to buy a notebook in which to make notes during sessions, record homework assignments, complete written assignments like monitoring or thought records, and jot down questions or concerns to ask the clinician.

In addition to session notes, the client's chart should also include records of all contacts with clients or other individuals involved in the case. If a client calls to discuss something with the clinician, a note should be made in the chart of the date and time of the call and what was discussed. If a client sends an e-mail to the clinician, this should be printed out and placed in the chart (along with the clinician's reply). Similarly, if the clinician speaks to other professionals involved in the case or to family members or friends of the client, these conversations should be documented.

FIGURE 8.1. Sample progress note for Michael, Session 2.

Name: Michael J.
Session No.: 2
Axis I: Social phobia
Axis II: Not assessed
Clinician: Dr. T.
Date: November 4, 2004

Session Goals and Objective: Complete psychoeducation and develop the fear and avoidance hierarchy.

Data

Homework from last session: Michael completed all of his homework, which consisted of monitoring the three components of anxiety in stressful social situations. Notably, Michael typed his homework and included a great deal of detail, suggesting that he might have been concerned with being negatively evaluated for not doing the homework perfectly.

Functional impairment: Michael had a very busy week with schoolwork, volunteering at a church soup kitchen, and leading a service on Sunday morning for some local college students. He was able to complete all of these tasks, but not without distress. On Saturday night, he stayed up very late rehearsing his sermon and felt very tired in church on Sunday morning. This week, Michael also had to complete a group project for one of his classes. He did a great deal of the work for the project, but asked his fellow group members to do the entire oral presentation. Michael made this decision despite knowing that it would affect his grade.

Current issues/topics/stressors: As noted above, social anxiety caused Michael a significant amount of distress this past week. While he was able to go about his usual activities, he experienced a lot of distress associated with them. He did, however, enjoy working at the soup kitchen and reported having some nice conversations with the people who dropped by for meals.

Interventions: In today's session, we reviewed the educational material covered in the session last week and finished going over the remaining material, which mostly consisted of a discussion of possible causes for social anxiety. Throughout psychoeducation, Michael exhibited a clear understanding of the CBT approach to treating social anxiety. During the remainder of the session, we developed Michael's hierarchy. Michael took a copy of the hierarchy home with him and was asked to add additional items that he would like to work on.

Observations: Michael seems to be on board with the treatment program. He expressed concern about the amount of time he had spent preparing for his sermon this week and also reported that he felt very angry with himself after getting out of speaking during his class presentation. He reported that he was looking forward to learning how to better deal with these situations.

Other: None.

(*continued on next page*)

FIGURE 8.1. (*continued*)

Assessment

The initial two sessions of therapy have gone well. Michael clearly understands the CBT approach and is eager to start using CBT techniques to work on his social anxiety.

Plan

- Continue to monitor the three components of anxiety in the upcoming week.
- Add items to hierarchy, if needed.
- Begin cognitive restructuring next week.

Time started: 4 P.M.   *Time finished:* 5 P.M.   *Duration:* 1 hour

Next appointment: November 11, 2004, 4 P.M.

Clinician's Signature: _____

Supervisor's Signature: _____

Chapter 9

■ ■ ■

MANAGING CLIENT NONCOMPLIANCE IN COGNITIVE-BEHAVIORAL THERAPY

In this chapter, we focus on the problem of client noncompliance or resistance in CBT. CBT is a structured approach to treatment, so there is a clear expectation that clients will engage in specific tasks in order to improve their functioning. Depending on the focus of treatment, such tasks might involve completing thought records, doing exposure exercises both during and outside of sessions, or changing specific behaviors like drinking or binge eating. *Noncompliance* is defined as an unwillingness to engage in the activities that clinicians know to be integral to good treatment outcome. With this definition in mind, it is obvious that client noncompliance can be a major roadblock in CBT (for a much more detailed discussion of these issues, see Robert L. Leahy's [2001] book *Overcoming Resistance in Cognitive Therapy*). Even the most skilled clinicians have difficulty working with clients who are not willing to do their part in therapy. Clinicians leave such sessions feeling exhausted, as if they did all of the work. Sessions might be spent convincing the client of the rationale, bargaining about certain assignments, or discussing very rigidly held beliefs. Given the active nature of CBT, most therapy sessions feel like hard work, but there is certainly a difference between feeling as if you and the client are climbing a mountain together and feeling as if you are climbing up the mountain dragging the client behind you.

Before attributing all difficult sessions to client noncompliance, however, give some thought to where you are in the therapy process. There is no doubt that clinicians take a more active role early on in treatment. During psychoeducation, even if you effectively involve the client, you will be doing most of the talking. Early in cognitive work, you will actively help clients identify their automatic thoughts and engage in cognitive restructuring. When first doing behavioral exercises, you might be the one to decide what these exercises will be. This is not at all to say that clients are not involved. They will, however, need a great deal of guidance.

In the middle stages of therapy, once clients have grasped the core concepts of CBT, they should start to take a more active role in the therapy. As they do so, they will be on their way to becoming their own therapists. Some clients will take to this role very well, and you will feel hopeful that they will continue to make progress once they are no longer seeing you.

Other clients will pose a much greater challenge. In our opinion, the way that noncompliance is perceived by the therapist can make a large difference. Rather than seeing it as a frustration and annoyance, view it with curiosity and use it to inform the case conceptualization. Try to figure out what is driving the noncompliance, and then try to come up with a clever solution to working around the roadblocks that you identify. Keeping this emotional distance from the problematic behavior will have a clear advantage with respect to the therapeutic relationship—rather than taking it personally, you place the focus on how to help the client. Therapy can be extremely rewarding when a noncompliant client engages in the treatment and ends up having success. In the sections that follow, we discuss two roadblocks that can be manifested as client noncompliance and offer recommendations for moving past them and continuing with the course of therapy.

ROADBLOCK 1: DIFFICULTIES WITH GETTING THE CLIENT TO ENGAGE IN THE PROCESS OF CBT

For CBT to work effectively, clients must see this approach as viable, and they must be willing to engage in the core techniques of the therapy. Clients who do not "buy" the CBT approach or who may not be motivated to change for one reason or another might start exhibiting various behaviors that interfere in the therapy process. Recognizing these behaviors, and knowing how to resolve them, are essential skills for the CBT clinician to acquire and hone.

Clients Who Repeatedly Miss Sessions or Come Late

Some clients frequently miss sessions without canceling in advance, ask to change session times on a frequent basis, or come to sessions late.

These clients might be very fearful of CBT or might doubt their ability to change. By not coming to sessions at all, clients can avoid the hard work of therapy. Coming late can also be seen as an example of avoidance behavior—the session time that is remaining when clients finally arrive is often spent discussing their lateness. The hard work of therapy is put off until the following session. Missing sessions and coming late can also be seen as self-handicapping strategies. If clients do not do the work of therapy, they cannot feel bad about themselves if it does not work effectively for them.

Solving the Problem

It would be a disservice to both clinician and client to bend to the pressures exerted by clients in these situations. Absenteeism and lateness, from the clinician's perspective, are terribly frustrating. For the first several minutes, we still expect the client to arrive and have a difficult time engaging in another task that we will just have to stop when the client finally appears. Once it becomes clear that the client is not coming, it feels as if there is not enough time left in the hour to do anything productive before the next client arrives. When clients arrive late, the clinician might come to feel resentful for being made to "wait around" and for not being able to carry out the session as planned. With clients who are repeatedly late, clinicians might feel bitter about having to spend session time talking about tardiness once again. These sessions are particularly anxiety-provoking for beginning clinicians, who can feel that they are being denied the experience of doing good therapy and who also worry about their supervisors' reactions to their clients being repeatedly absent or late. Obviously, absenteeism and lateness take away from the benefits that clients could derive from therapy.

A good place to start is by asking clients directly why they were late or missed a session. Some will come right out and say, "I did not want to do that exposure we had planned for today" or "I ended up getting really drunk last night and didn't wake up in time for our session." When clients are frank in this way, their concerns can be dealt with directly. When clients say that they do not know why they behaved the way they did, clinicians can offer them some possible explanations.

Clients should be asked if they were nervous about what was supposed to be happening in the session that day or if they had a negative experience with what occurred in the previous session. They should also be asked if their thoughts about treatment or about their ability to make positive changes got in the way. For example, clients can be asked, "Are you worried that the treatment isn't going to help you?" Finally, clients should be asked if their tardiness or absenteeism is related to the presenting problem for which they are seeking treatment. A depressed client may have trouble getting motivated to come to sessions, or a client with OCD may be delayed at home by rituals. Other clients might be too anxious to tell you that a particular meeting time is not working well for them.

The goal of these questions is to determine what is standing in the way of clients' timely and regular attendance. Once we identify the obstacles, cognitive and behavioral techniques can be used to help clients work through them. For example, a client who had difficulty with assertiveness, and therefore had a hard time telling the clinician that the established time for sessions was inconvenient for him, was assigned the task of calling the clinician a few times during the week to repeatedly change the session time. Although this was slightly annoying for the clinician, it turned out to be a very effective exercise for the client. Once the client had accomplished this task, a new session time agreeable to both clinician and client was set. They then designed a number of additional in-session and homework exercises to continue practicing assertiveness.

One last issue deserves mention. Beginning clinicians are often worried about being well liked by their clients. Therefore, they tend to be overly flexible about rebooking appointments, seeing clients when they arrive even if they are very late, and so on. Although most clients will from time to time miss an appointment or come late to session, bending to the requests of clients who are chronically late or regularly miss sessions does them no favors. Keep in mind that clients' behaviors in therapy are a window into their lives outside of therapy, and these clients likely have the same problems with work, social commitments, and other appointments. Although we, as clinicians, might be understanding of such behaviors, others in clients' "real worlds" are unlikely to be as generous. With this in mind, therapy is the perfect venue for helping clients to see the negative effects of their lateness and absenteeism on others and on themselves.

Clients Who Are Resistant to In-Session Work

Even for more seasoned clinicians, it is always an interesting experience when clients continue to come to therapy sessions regularly but steadfastly refuse to do most of what is suggested to them. It is almost as if the client would like the clinician to wave a magic wand and make all of their problems disappear. As with clients prone to absenteeism or lateness, clinicians may understandably believe that they are wasting their time with such clients, and they might feel resentful that clients who actually would make an effort in therapy are waiting for treatment while places are taken up by ones who are making no effort whatsoever. Although these situations are undoubtedly frustrating, it is essential to try to figure out what is blocking the client's progress.

Solving the Problem

Fear and uncertainty are very often obstacles for clients who come to therapy and do not do the required work. In this section, we discuss how to move clients beyond these roadblocks, but before doing so one caveat is worth mentioning. From time to time, clients will come to therapy and refuse to do work because the simple act of being physically present at sessions provides significant reward for them. Monetary gain or other benefits (e.g., having one's spouse believe that one is "making an effort") might be more important to the client than actual change. It is important to remember that clinicians have no obligation to treat clients who will not engage in treatment, and it would be unethical to complete paperwork (e.g., for disability) saying that clients are truly engaged in treatment when they are not.

With that being said, let us to return to the more common scenario—clients feeling worried about what will happen if they engage in CBT. A good starting point is to simply ask clients what they fear—sometimes they will reveal fears that are completely irrational and that can be corrected through simple psychoeducation and the use of cognitive-behavioral techniques. Many clients with eating disorders, for example, fear that if they begin to eat "normally" they will gain weight and that their weight will then escalate indefinitely (e.g., a person who weighs 100 pounds will quickly weigh 300 pounds). One client of ours who had panic disorder was afraid that if she experienced panic symptoms, she might never "come out of it" and might end up becoming "psychotic." The client believed that this would land her in the locked ward of a mental hospital for the rest of her life. Rather than risk this outcome, the client rarely left her house—the one place where she did not experience panic symptoms. Brief psychoeducation can be used to teach clients that while normal eating might lead to some weight gain, it is unlikely that weight gain will never cease. Similarly, there is no evidence to suggest that panic symptoms lead to psychosis. For some clients, psychoeducation is sufficient to ameliorate their fears and facilitate their engagement with therapy.

For others, psychoeducation will not be enough. The conundrum is that the best way to dispel clients' faulty beliefs is through direct experience. For example, by normalizing eating, clients will learn that weight will not increase indefinitely. Similarly, by inducing panic symptoms, the client will learn that she will not become psychotic and that she can actually cope with the symptoms quite well. However, selling this rationale to clients can sometimes be difficult. One helpful tool is to remind clients that changes in CBT are made relatively gradually. Although they must make *some* changes right from the start of therapy, clients are encouraged to build on their experiences in CBT—tackling increasingly difficult tasks as they gain a sense of self-efficacy and are able to dispel some of their dysfunctional beliefs.

Another tool that we have found useful is getting clients to think about how they would feel if they accomplished a difficult task. Clients sometimes like to think in terms of analogies that are removed from their own issue of concern. A helpful example is exercising. Very few of us leap out of bed at 6 A.M. to exercise. A good motivating tactic at that hour of the day is reminding yourself how you will feel when it is over. If we do not exercise, we might spend the day regretting it; if we do, it is unlikely that we will have any thoughts except positive ones.

The client who was scared of having a psychotic break due to her panic symptoms was asked how she would feel if she were able to take her children to school one day. Her immediate response was that it would be terrifying. She was then asked, "But what if you were able to do it and your feared outcomes did not occur?" This client, who had never before taken her young children to school, looked at the clinician almost in awe and responded, "That would feel so amazing." The idea of this feeling of accomplishment was incredibly motivating to the client, and, throughout treatment, she often reminded herself of how good she would feel once difficult tasks were accomplished.

On a more long-term scale, it is also useful to help clients conduct a cost–benefit analysis. Do the potential benefits of treatment outweigh the costs of doing the treatment? Inevitably, clients recognize that the potential gains will outweigh the potential losses. One problem that we sometimes encounter is that clients do not know what they would like to gain. Some clients come in to therapy with a very clear picture of what life would be like when they no longer have the difficulties that are causing them so much distress and impairment. Perhaps they want to spend more time with their children, start dating, go back to school, or get a desired job. Articulating these desires can be very powerful for clients and can be used as a "hook" to draw them back in when they are resistant to a particular intervention.

Some clients have more difficulty articulating these "What would life be like . . . " scenarios. This often occurs with clients with very long-standing difficulties, who perhaps do not have a good baseline of functioning to which they would like to return. With these clients, it is worth spending some time establishing goals and doing some problem solving about how to accomplish them. For example, for a client who has not worked in his or her adult life, a referral for vocational counseling might be helpful. Assisting the client in formulating some long-term goals can be very motivating during treatment.

To summarize, clients who keep coming to sessions but refuse to do the work of treatment are indeed perplexing. This behavior, while frustrating to the clinician, indicates that the client wishes to change, but that something is standing in the way. It is our job to uncover what that roadblock is. In some cases it is fear, and you can use CBT techniques to help clients work past it. In other cases the difficulties lie in the client's motivation to change. Helping clients to see what life would be like once they have made some difficult changes can be a very positive step in the therapy process.

Clients Who Use Diversionary Tactics

Some clients come to therapy and are more than willing to work, but they are always trying to put off working on the problem for which they sought treatment. This most often presents itself in the form of clients who seem to experience a new stressful event every week. Take, for example, a client who presented for treatment of panic disorder with agoraphobia. When the therapy program was introduced, the client felt a great deal of trepidation about the idea of exposing himself to feared situations and symptoms. At the time in treatment when exposures were about to begin, the client started to have weekly crises. One week, he had broken up with his girlfriend, the next week he had had an argument with a coworker, and the next he was feeling very worried about his mother, who was about to have surgery. This client came into sessions wanting to discuss these stressful events, rather than focusing on his panic disorder. This scenario can throw beginning clinicians a curveball. On one hand, there is often pressure to stick to the treatment goal (helping the client to deal with his panic attacks). On the other hand, a clinician can come across as lacking empathy if he or she constantly pushes the client's other difficulties aside.

Solving the Problem

It is very important to examine the nature of the relationship between stressors and the presenting problem, since they are often related in some meaningful way. Helping clients to recognize these connections will support the clinician's desire to keep the therapy on track:

CLINICIAN: Tom, do you see any connection between what's been going on in your life these last few weeks and your panic symptoms?

TOM: Well, all this stress is certainly making me have more panic attacks.

CLINICIAN: That's an important observation. Any thoughts on how the relationship might work in the other direction? Has panic played any role in the stressors you've been experiencing?

TOM: What do you mean?

CLINICIAN: Well, let's start with the first difficult situation you had a few weeks ago when Ann broke up with you. Did panic have anything to do with that?

TOM: Of course. I mean, Ann was just sick of all of it. Look at me—I can't go to movies, I can't travel, I can't go to the gym. These were things we used to do all the time. And now I am this bundle of nerves who can't do anything.

CLINICIAN: How about the conflict at work?

TOM: Mary was furious at me. We were working on a project together, and I missed work for the 2 days before it was due. I got up on the wrong side of the bed. Right from when I got out of bed, I was anxious and I just knew if I went to work, I'd be panicking all day. Mary was left to finish up the whole project.

CLINICIAN: So again, you can see a pretty clear connection between your panic disorder and these stressors.

TOM: I guess.

CLINICIAN: So, each week, you've been wanting to come in and talk about these stressful things that happened. Given what we've just discussed, is there another way we might be able to tackle your problems?

TOM: I don't know. All I can think about when I come in here is how upset I am about what's gone wrong during the week.

CLINICIAN: What about preventing more stressful things from going on the following week?

TOM: Don't I wish.

CLINICIAN: Well, let's think about this. If panic is playing a pretty direct role in some of these interpersonal situations, what would happen if we worked on the panic?

TOM: Oh. So, you're saying that if I had worked on my panic, Ann wouldn't have broken up with me and Mary wouldn't have been furious at me and life would be perfect?

CLINICIAN: There is no way to know that, and we can't change what has already happened. But what about thinking more in terms of when you start dating new women or doing better at work the next time you have a group presentation?

TOM: You're saying that if the panic is better, I'd have an easier time of it.

CLINICIAN: Do you think you would?

TOM: Well, right now, no woman is going to date me. I can barely leave the house. And, yeah, I'm already dreading my next presentation at work.

CLINICIAN: Is it worth trying for a few weeks to stay really focused on the panic and see how that rubs off on life outside of our sessions?

TOM: So, you mean getting out there and doing those exposures?

CLINICIAN: Yes, that's what I mean.

TOM: I don't want to, but what else can I do?

Sometimes the connections between life stressors and the presenting problem are not as clear, and sometimes there is no connection at all. There are two possible outcomes in such cases. When clients are in therapy, their lives outside of therapy continue and pressing issues do come up. It can be appropriate to shift focus away from the presenting problem for a time to put out these "fires." This might be the case when a problem is so upsetting that it makes it hard to focus on anything else (e.g., the breakup of a marriage, the death of a loved one) or when the need to solve a problem is time-sensitive (e.g., needing to decide whether or not to accept a job offer by a certain deadline). In such cases, the client and the clinician should agree on the number of sessions that will be dedicated to working on the crisis, at which time the focus will be shifted back to the presenting problem.

Other clients come in to therapy with crises "du jour," so to speak—new problems all the time, which do not seem particularly significant or pressing. Clinicians should consider whether these clients are trying to avoid the "real" problem for which they sought treatment, simply because it is too frightening. Consider our client with panic disorder at the session following his first exposure session:

TOM: I just want you to know that things have not been better since we rode the subway last week. I am so stressed about my mom and I want to talk about that today.

CLINICIAN: Can you tell me what you mean when you say that "things have not been better"?

TOM: I had a bunch of panic attacks this week. So it doesn't make me really want to go and do a whole bunch of other stuff.

CLINICIAN: Let's think for a second about the goals that we set for this week. Do you remember what they were?

TOM: I think I wrote them down in my notebook. I can't really remember.

CLINICIAN: Well, let's take a look.

TOM: It says here that my goal was to ride the subway 3 times this week.

CLINICIAN: And?

TOM: I didn't do it. I was so nervous. I was having all these panic attacks and knew if I went on the subway, I'd have one for sure.

CLINICIAN: Okay, let's look at a few things here. How was it when we rode the subway together last week?

TOM: Fine.

CLINICIAN: Just fine?

TOM: I was really excited after our session last week. I hadn't been on the subway since high school.

CLINICIAN: What was our goal for that exposure?

TOM: Just to ride the subway. You wouldn't let me set the goal of riding the subway and not panicking.

CLINICIAN: Why?

TOM: Well, because you said what mattered was doing it, not how it felt.

CLINICIAN: So, whether or not you had a panic attack was not important.

TOM: I wouldn't say it wasn't important!

CLINICIAN: Right. I meant that it wasn't important to the outcome of the exposure.

TOM: Right.

CLINICIAN: So, what do you think would have happened if you had gone on the subway this week?

TOM: I might have had a panic attack.

CLINICIAN: You might have. Could that still have been a useful experience?

TOM: I guess. I suppose the idea is to see that I can manage the attacks when they do happen.

CLINICIAN: Right. So, let me ask you this. If you had gone on the subway this week and had some positive experiences, do you think you would feel differently about what we should do in today's session?

TOM: Maybe. I guess if I worked on the subway this week and felt that I dealt with it well, I would be ready to do the next thing in our session today.

CLINICIAN: That's an interesting thought. With that in mind, what do you think would be useful for us to do today?

TOM: Well, we were going to go in an elevator in a tall building. Maybe we could take the subway there and practice that a bit more. So, we could do two things today.

CLINICIAN: I think that's a great idea. And let's leave some time at the end of our session to talk about how your mom is doing and how to cope with some of the stress you're experiencing with that situation.

TOM: Sounds good.

In summary, there are various ways to manage clients who make use of diversionary tactics. The most important point is to try to work through with clients *why* they are diverting attention from the problem that was meant to be the focus of treatment. Sometimes the issues that are most problematic to clients do shift over time, necessitating flexibility in the therapy. At other times, clients use other issues as a means of avoiding working on the main problem, often failing to recognize the connections between multiple issues in their lives. Helping clients to see these connections can be beneficial for getting the therapy back on track. One final point to keep in mind is that we should not shut down our clients completely every time they bring up an issue that does not fit with the plan for therapy. This communicates to clients a lack of empathy, understanding, and compassion. Rather, work other issues into the agenda so that some time is left for them (and to evaluate whether more time should be committed to them), without allowing the therapy to get terribly off track.

Clients Who Resist Homework

Although many clients initially balk at the idea of once again having homework in their lives, many are quite agreeable to do it once they understand the rationale underlying it. Unfortunately, good intentions do not always translate into doing, and you will become all too familiar with clients who come to sessions not having done their homework. Failure to do homework can result from many different factors, and it is important to understand what happened in order to achieve better compliance with homework in the future.

Solving the Problem

Difficulties involving homework noncompliance can be the responsibility of the client, but they can also be attributed to the clinician. Before considering the role played by clients, it is important to emphasize what clinicians need to do to encourage homework compliance. Clinicians often let homework slip through the cracks. They might forget to assign homework at the end of a session, or they might assign it but forget to review it at the beginning of the next session. This makes clients believe that homework is not important to the treatment and will likely lead to noncompliance in the future.

Session agendas are very helpful for managing this problem. Make sure to leave enough time at the end of the session to assign homework. Encourage clients to record their homework assignments in writing to serve as a reminder of what they need to do during the week. You should also record their assignment, and the first agenda item in the next session should be to return to that list and discuss each item on it.

Another difficulty that clinicians have is taking too much control over the assignment of homework. Early on in therapy, it is appropriate for the clinician to design the homework. Later on, this task should shift to the client. Although the clinician should obviously serve as a guide in this process, clients will be more likely to complete homework assignments if they design them. Along these same lines, homework assignments should be relevant to clients' concerns. If a client with panic disorder and agoraphobia lives in a small town outside a big city and rarely needs to go into the city, it might not be useful for the clinician to assign as homework riding on the subway or taking an elevator to the top of a tall building. Rather, the client might tell the clinician that she would like to visit her local supermarket and take her children to the library. Not only will clients be more likely to comply with homework assignments that are relevant to them, but they will also gain much more from the treatment in terms of improved functioning in their everyday lives.

A final difficulty that clinicians sometimes have is failing to adequately reinforce clients for doing homework. Although it is certainly important for clients to feel inherently good about having done homework, receiving encouragement from the clinician can also go a long way. Clinicians sometimes need to be cheerleaders for the very hard work that their clients do.

Homework noncompliance can also stem from client-related factors. One of the most common reasons that clients will give for homework noncompliance is a lack of time. Beginning clinicians, wanting to be empathic to their clients, can fall into the trap of accepting this as an excuse. This does a disservice to clients. Homework is an essential part of CBT—the more time that clients commit to working on their difficulties, the more likely it is that they will make positive gains during treatment.

The "I didn't have time" excuse should be dealt with early in therapy. One solution is to help clients work through the process of planning when and how to do their homework. This seems quite simple, but it can be a substantial roadblock for many clients. They might be overwhelmed with so many other things in their lives that it is hard to put plans into action. For example, our client, Tom, who had panic disorder, could have been helped to plan for doing his subway exposures in the week following the subway ride he took in session with his clinician. If Tom walked to work in order to avoid the subway, he and his clinician could have worked out a plan for him to ride the subway each day that week. In this way, he would not have to set aside separate times for homework per se. Instead, he would have worked it into his already busy schedule and actually saved time by getting to work faster!

Homework cannot always be so gracefully integrated into clients' days. Rather, they need to see how important it is to make time for homework, in much the same way that they would make time to call a friend, pay their bills, or go to the gym. For clients who have a great deal going on in their lives, they might actually have to put some other activities on hold during therapy in order to have time to commit to their homework. If clients are resistant to making adequate time for homework, a good strategy is to return to the rationale and review with clients why homework is so important to the therapy process. There is no doubt that CBT is hard work, and clinicians must emphasize to clients that change will not come about without effort. At the same time, however, clients should be encouraged to reward themselves for doing homework. Clients might choose to reward themselves with a favorite food (e.g., "After I do this homework assignment, I am going to have a chocolate chip cookie") or activity (e.g., "Once I do my thought records, I am going to watch my favorite TV show"). Some clients with whom we have worked have planned a special reward for themselves once therapy is complete such as going on a weekend trip or buying some new clothes.

Another roadblock to homework compliance, which can be attributable to the clinician and/or the client, is assigning homework that is too difficult or too time-consuming. Some clients will tell their clinicians that this was the problem; others will say that they did not have time to do homework, but with some probing will admit that this was the real reason. Early in therapy, we want our clients to have positive experiences. We want them to see that they can manage the treatment and that doing the treatment can have a positive effect. Therefore, if clients complain early in treatment that they were assigned too much homework or that the homework assignments were too hard, it would be appropriate to make some alterations. Do not cut out homework altogether, just assign something that is more manageable. Although the assignment might seem overly simple, succeeding at a homework assignment will increase the likelihood that the client will complete future homework assignments. Later in therapy, clients should be encouraged to take a more active role in designing homework assignments. Sometimes clients "bite off more than they can chew," and feel ashamed to report that they did not accomplish what they had planned. Ideally, the clinician will recognize such a problem as the homework assignment is being designed. If this does not happen and clients report "failure" at the next session, the clinician can help them to identify the factors that prevented them from doing the homework and design an assignment for the next week that takes these factors into account.

Finally, some clients avoid doing homework because they are worried about doing it incorrectly and being judged negatively by the clinician. The best way to deal with this potential problem is to ward it off right from the start of treatment. The very first time that homework is assigned, let clients know that a lot of other clients worry that you will judge them based on their homework and that this prevents some clients from doing homework at all. Tell clients that you are there to teach them new skills and not to judge them. This is a message that should be repeated regularly throughout treatment.

Another way to prevent this problem is to be mindful of your reactions to clients' homework. Often, clients do not do homework exactly as we had hoped, particularly early in treatment. Although it is very important to fix mistakes, it is even more important to not damage rapport. If you would like to correct something that a client has done, first reinforce him or her for what has been done and then gently make some suggestions for improvements on the next assignment.

A Final Issue to Consider:
Are Clients Afraid of a Life without Psychological Problems?

Some clients come to therapy seemingly eager to make changes, but do very little to move themselves in that direction. They might not come to sessions, they might come late, and, when they do come, they might be highly resistant to our suggestions. Clinicians should always consider whether clients are nervous about making changes in their lives—mostly because of what life will hold for them once they have resolved their difficulties. As we noted earlier, some clients have a very clear vision of what life will be like when they are no longer impaired by the difficulties that brought them in to therapy. This seems to be particularly true for clients who, at one time, were functioning very well. They might want to get back to a job that they loved, be able to spend more time with friends or family members, or perhaps try to accomplish new goals that were stymied by psychological problems. Other clients might not have something that they want to get back to per se, but might still be able to conjure up an image of a better life.

It is important to be aware that some clients who have suffered for a long time with psychological difficulties might feel as if they have missed out on life. They might look around and see that people with whom they grew up (friends, siblings, classmates) have accomplished things in life that they have not been able to accomplish. For example, a client's sibling might have bought a home, married, had children, and established a career. For a client who, at least in part because of psychological problems, has remained single, lost friends, not established a career, and struggled financially, this comparison can be devastating. Furthermore, clients might feel that they have "missed the boat" and that it is now too late to achieve these things. This most certainly can decrease motivation to work hard in treatment—after all, the light at the end of the tunnel is not particularly bright.

Clinicians should be careful to observe these stated beliefs among their clients. They are most likely to emerge when asking clients about the costs and benefits of doing treatment and, related to this, how they picture their lives once therapy is over. Such concerns about "missing the boat" should be incorporated into therapy by helping clients to articulate what they feel they have missed and using problem-solving strategies to close these gaps. For example, if clients fear that at the end of therapy, they will not be able to support themselves since they never established a career, you might want to discuss career-related issues with them or refer them to a vocational counselor. Similarly, you might want to incorporate into therapy ways that clients can meet new friends or potential romantic partners. The idea is to use cognitive and behavioral techniques to help clients move past the barriers that they perceive to be standing in the way of accomplishing these important goals.

ROADBLOCK 2: CLIENT DIFFICULTIES WITH THE THERAPEUTIC RELATIONSHIP

Often, clients have grown up with very critical families, in families where it was unacceptable to express emotion, or in homes where it was shameful to have psychological difficulties. As adults, they might have tried to seek help and support from significant others and, as in their earlier lives, might have been rebuffed. People in their lives might have not wanted to be "dragged down" by their problems or might have had difficulties understanding their problems. Some clients do get support from significant others in their lives, but often their advice is not helpful (e.g., "Just snap out of it"). As a result of these experiences, clients come to therapy with the expectation that clinicians will react to them in much the same way as have the other people in their lives. In other words, they may expect that they will not be understood or supported. They might expect that nothing the clinician can tell them will help. These expectations can lead clients to behave in ways that have a negative impact on the therapeutic process. As noted earlier, rather than reacting negatively to therapy-interfering behaviors, we should consider them with curiosity, figure out how they might be related to clients' lives, and try to help clients behave within the therapeutic environment in a way that would be more conducive to our work with them.

"My Client Will Not Open Up"

Despite our best efforts to put clients at ease and make them feel comfortable about sharing their difficulties, some clients will be very reluctant to open up. Some clients might talk quite a bit, but you might be left with the sense that they are not being completely forthcoming about their difficulties. They might answer your questions with a single word or give only the most basic information. Some clients refuse to answer certain questions completely. This can make therapy difficult, if not impossible.

Solving the Problem

The best way to deal with this problem is to be direct—but in an empathic way. First, make an observation to the client (e.g., "You seem reluctant to talk to me about these difficulties") and then pose an open-ended question (e.g., "What are your concerns?"). Asking close-ended questions (e.g., "Are you feeling uncomfortable?") with resistant clients is not a good strategy, because they promote the continued use of one-word answers.

Why might clients be reluctant to share personal information with their clinicians? Some clients worry about confidentiality. They might have had negative experiences with clinicians before or might have felt violated by other people in their lives (e.g., a sibling sharing private information with a parent). Although the issue of confidentiality is covered with clients very early in our interactions with them, it can be very helpful with reticent clients to reiterate your concern for confidentiality and the efforts that you take to ensure it.

Another common client concern is that they will be negatively evaluated by the clinician because of the difficulties that they are having. This fear might exist for good reason—they might have shared their difficulties with significant others in the past and indeed have been negatively evaluated. Some clients are so scared of being judged negatively that they have never before shared their problems with anyone. Therefore, they will have gained no evidence to refute their contention that the reaction of others will be negative when they do share.

What exactly do clients fear? Taking a broad perspective, some clients have been judged negatively by others in their lives simply because they have mental health problems. Being in therapy means that clients have admitted that they have a mental health problem and that they need help. This might be very hard for clients who were raised to believe that mental health problems are a sign of weakness or who have significant others who hold this belief. In such cases, cognitive restructuring can be used to help clients to view their situation in a different light. Although some people might view seeking therapy as a sign of weakness, it can certainly also be seen as a sign of courage. Clients have decided to undertake very hard work in order to better their lives. Viewing therapy in this way is much more positive and motivating than seeing it as a sign of weakness.

On a more specific level, some clients might have received critical feedback for the kind of symptoms that they have. They might have been labeled by others (or feared being labeled by others) as odd, unusual, or crazy. Clients may then fear that revealing their symptoms to clinicians will yield these same reactions. Often, clients will comment to this effect: "I can't really tell you what's going on—you'll think I'm a complete nut" or "I'm not going to tell you everything about my problem—I'm sure you've never met another client who's going through what I'm going through." In these situations, it is important to let clients know that you are there to help them and not to judge them. The best evidence for this will come when they do begin to reveal information and see that your reaction is supportive, noncritical, and empathic.

Significant others in clients' lives might have also made them feel bad about the origins of their problems and/or their ability to "fix their problems." Consider the case of a young woman named Jane who presented for treatment of posttraumatic stress disorder (PTSD) 5 years after having been raped. During treatment, Jane was extremely reluctant to share the details of her story with the clinician.

CLINICIAN: You seem to be having a hard time letting me in on what happened.

JANE: Yeah. It's harder than I thought it would be.

CLINICIAN: Had you ever told anyone else about what happened?

JANE: Two people. And boy, was that an (*sarcastically*) excellent experience.

CLINICIAN: Can you tell me about that?

JANE: Well, like I've already told you, I was raped by a guy I barely knew when I was in college. A few days after it happened, I told my roommate. It was not a good thing at all.

CLINICIAN: How did she react?

JANE: Well, she told me I asked for it.

CLINICIAN: That must have been really hard for you, especially so soon after it happened.

JANE: You must be thinking the same thing. I mean, don't you agree that going home with a guy you barely know is asking for trouble?

CLINICIAN: I don't think any woman ever "asks to be raped."

JANE: Well, I probably did ask for it. I went on one date with this guy, he invited me back to his frat house and, after one drink, raped me.

CLINICIAN: It must have been very difficult for you to go through such a frightening experience and then not find any support or help from a friend.

JANE: The other time I tried wasn't so good either.

CLINICIAN: When was that?

JANE: About 3 years ago. I never dated for the rest of college. Three years ago, I finally started dating and met this guy I really liked. But, whenever we got intimate, I'd freak out and say I wasn't ready. I just felt like there was so much about me that he didn't understand.

CLINICIAN: So, you told him about the rape?

JANE: I did. And, you know what he said?

CLINICIAN: What?

JANE: He told me that it was 3 years ago and to snap out of it. He just didn't get how something like that could still be bothering me so much.

CLINICIAN: I am sorry you've had such negative experiences with trying to get help. I am really glad that you've come to see me. But, it seems that maybe these bad experiences have colored how you feel about being here too. Am I hearing that correctly?

JANE: I am just at a point where I don't trust anyone. I just think that anyone I tell is going to think that it was my fault and that if I was making more effort now, I'd have moved past all of this.

CLINICIAN: You've just told me part of the story of what happened to you and I am not having that reaction at all. Quite the opposite, in fact.

JANE: What do you mean?

CLINICIAN: Well, we work with a lot of women here who have been raped. I have yet to meet one who has asked for that to happen to her. And I have seen many women who have tried for years to move on and just can't do it on their own. I think a very brave thing to do is to come and get some help.

JANE: So, you're trying to say that I should feel okay talking about this stuff with you?

CLINICIAN: I don't like telling clients how they "should" feel. All I can tell you is that the reaction I am having to you right now is very different from how it sounds like your roommate and ex-boyfriend reacted to you. Given those experiences, I can see your reluctance. But I hope that you'll come to feel comfortable here and believe that you can share things without being judged.

JANE: I think I'm okay with telling you a bit more.

In summary, when dealing with clients who are reluctant to share much, the first thing that the clinician should do is try to figure out what clients fear will happen if they do share. Are they afraid that their confidentiality will be breached? Are they scared that the clinician will see them as weak or crazy? Are they nervous that the clinician will react in an unhelpful, accusatory way like others might have reacted toward them in the past? Once clinicians help clients to articulate these concerns, we can help them to see that the therapeutic relationship is unique, based on support and empathy, rather than negative judgment.

"My Client Talks Too Much"

On the other end of the spectrum, we meet clients who want to share everything with us. Clients of this sort can be particularly challenging when we are using highly structured assessment measures (e.g., structured interviews) or therapeutic interventions (e.g., CBT). Containing talkative clients can be very difficult. Therapy is premised on clients being able to self-disclose, yet sharing a great deal of extraneous information is typically counterproductive. Furthermore, when clients barrage us with a great deal of information, it can be difficult to extract the information that is important and most salient to treatment.

Solving the Problem

As in the case of clients who are hesitant to talk, when dealing with clients who talk too much, we should be direct and try to uncover why clients are having difficulties with succinctness. One simple explanation, particularly during the process of assessment, is that clients simply don't know what is expected of them in the therapeutic setting. They likely don't know that therapists ask questions in a particular way to get the information that they need to conceptualize the case and develop appropriate interventions. Without this knowledge, they might feel pressure to provide lots of details to make sure the clinician understands the problems they are facing. It is fine for clinicians to acknowledge this and reassure clients that there is a framework to their questioning. For example, they can say, "In today's session, I am going to be asking you about all sorts of issues that can pose problems for you. Some of them might apply, in which case we'll spend more time discussing them, and some might not, in which case we'll move on. At the end of the evaluation, I'll ask you if we've missed anything important. So, there will be ample opportunity at the end of our session to make sure I have a good understanding of your problems." This type of introduction gives clients a framework for the session, and reassures them that they can "fill in the blanks" at the end of the session if anything pertinent was overlooked.

Another common reason for chattiness is anxiety. A lot of people (including those without any psychological disorders) are aware that when they feel anxious, they begin to chatter incessantly. You might notice that some clients are very chatty in the first session or two of treatment and then start to speak more appropriately. Similarly, some clients are chatty at the beginning of sessions and, as they settle in, they seem better able to contain themselves. For these clients, it might not be necessary to point out the problem since it quickly self-corrects when clients become acclimated to the clinician and the treatment.

Some clients will continue to be chatty even once you think that their anxiety should have habituated. These clients often get off on tangents, talking about all sorts of material that is not relevant to the treatment at hand. This can be viewed as a diversionary tactic, similar to the behavior of clients who repeatedly come to session with a new crisis. A good way to handle the problem is to leave a bit of time at the end of the session to "chat" in a less structured way, while dedicating the bulk of therapy time to dealing with the problem at hand in a more structured manner.

One final thing for clinicians to be aware of is that talkativeness can be related to specific psychological problems. For example, some clients with OCD are concerned with saying "just the right thing" or with providing totally complete information. They might repeat things that they already said in order to try to say it again "perfectly" or they might provide all sorts of extraneous information because they fear missing something. In these situations, clinicians should specifically point out the behavior to clients and explore whether it is related to the difficulties for which they are seeking treatment. If there is a relationship, talkativeness can be integrated into the treatment program. For example, the OCD client described earlier might work with the clinician to answer a series of increasingly complex questions with a single sentence.

"My Client Is Always Angry and Irritated"

Dealing with clients who are extremely critical, irritable, and angry can be very challenging to the clinician. Not surprisingly, beginning clinicians tend to personalize these client behaviors. They assume that the client must not like them or must be dissatisfied with the treatment. Some get very defensive and perhaps even verbally lash out at clients. Others, feeling very insulted, might be afraid of showing fear or even crying when a client lashes out. Neither of these reactions is particularly helpful in the context of the therapeutic relationship, even though they are genuine and likely mirror the reactions of others who deal with the client on a daily basis.

Solving the Problem

One of the best pieces of advice for beginning clinicians in these situations is to not get "sucked into" the anger. Instead, view it as another window into the client's life—one that can help you to conceptualize the case and develop interventions that will benefit the client in the "real world." Why might a client bring anger into the therapeutic relationship? One possibility is that clients feel desperate for help. They might have tried to improve their lives on their own with limited success. Perhaps they sought the help of others in their lives or of other mental health professional and these strategies were also unhelpful. Clients might fear that their situation is hopeless and that nothing that they try will make a difference. Some clients will simply reveal these concerns to clinicians—indeed, this is quite a good problem-solving strategy. Others might be less skilled at problem solving and might keep these concerns bottled up. When they feel frustrated, their frustration emerges as anger. When clients lash out at clinicians, one way to try to get at the thoughts that clients are having is to say "You seem very frustrated today. Can you help me to understand why?" Having frustration pointed out can be less threatening than having anger pointed out.

One should also consider how clients relate to other people in their lives. Clients who repeatedly get angry at clinicians might have grown up in homes where anger was frequently exhibited. As adults, they might have continued to be in interpersonal relationships where anger is a typical mode of relating. Simply put, clients might have developed a belief that others only hear them when they are angry.

Regardless of why clients are relating in an angry way, it is essential to deal with it. Clinicians should always know that they are in control of the tone in the therapy session. It is absolutely fine to let clients know what kind of behavior is unacceptable in therapy. This clinician could say, "I can see you are reluctant to do what I'm suggesting for our session today. I'd be fine discussing the issue with you further. What I am not fine with is yelling in therapy. I find it terribly counterproductive, and I am going to ask that there be no yelling in our sessions."

Ground rules like this can work wonders. For beginning clinicians, they communicate that, despite inexperience, the clinician is in charge of the session. For clients, being told that they will be heard without having to scream might be a very unique message. It can be a very powerful experience for clients to see that there are other modes of communication besides ones that are premised on anger and aggression.

Other clients will continue to have difficulties with anger expression even after efforts on the part of the clinician to curtail it. In these cases, the possibility of working on anger management within therapy sessions can be introduced. This is tricky, since few clients who exhibit difficulties with anger during therapy have actually presented for treatment of anger problems. Therefore, the clinician must introduce the issue with the client in a noncritical manner and find some "hook" that might make working on interpersonal issues more salient.

Consider a client named Jeff, who presented for CBT of depression. Early in therapy, the client was asked to complete daily thought records during the week. When the thought records were first introduced during a session, the client steadfastly refused to write anything down during therapy. He began to scream at his clinician, telling him that he had spent years in school and was certainly not going to start doing assignments again. The clinician was quite taken aback by the client's behavior. At first, he tried calmly to reiterate the rationale for the thought records—perhaps the client did not understand why they were so important. The client understood the rationale perfectly, but he still refused to do them, and he refused in a rude, aggressive way. In the next session, the following conversation ensued:

CLINICIAN: It seemed to me that you were pretty angry in last week's session when we spoke about the thought records. I thought we'd talk a bit about that in today's session. When was the last time you felt angry like that in your life outside of therapy?

JEFF: The last time? Gee, that's hard. I have a pretty bad temper in me, you know.

CLINICIAN: Well, let's think. Have you felt irritated with anyone or anything today?

JEFF: No. It's only 9 A.M., Doc. I'm doing okay so far.

CLINICIAN: Okay. How about yesterday?

JEFF: Yeah. That was a rough one. There were a few things. On the way to work, I was running really late, and the car in front of me was just creeping along. I was boiling inside. I was so mad at how slow this jerk was driving. We were on a one-way street, which technically holds one lane of traffic. But I was so mad, I just drove up next to him, gave him the finger and got in front of him. I was up on the curb; the road was so narrow.

CLINICIAN: What happened after that?

JEFF: Well, I was so fired up. I got to work and my secretary hadn't sent a fax I had left for her yesterday. I screamed my lungs out at her. She looked like she was about to cry her eyes out.

CLINICIAN: How did that make you feel?

JEFF: A little bad later on once I calmed down. I mean, the fax went out at 9:30 instead of 9:00. It didn't feel like a big deal once it had passed.

CLINICIAN: Did anything else happen yesterday?

JEFF: Gee, you think I've got a problem here, don't you?

CLINICIAN: What do you mean?

JEFF: You're accusing me.

CLINICIAN: Nope. It's just that I saw something in our session last week that made me wonder about how things are for you outside of our sessions. You got quite angry and in my view, that got in the way of having a productive session. I am just trying to see if that was an isolated incident—kind of a bad day, or if what I saw is something that happens for you often outside of sessions.

JEFF: Well, I stand accused then. I get ticked off *a lot*. What can you do?

CLINICIAN: What can we do?

JEFF: Well, I'm not here to learn to be less angry; I'm here to feel less depressed.

CLINICIAN: My concern from last week is that we'll have trouble working on your depression if anger and irritability continue to get in the way of our work together.

JEFF: What do you mean?

CLINICIAN: Do you think that the anger and depression fit together in any way?

JEFF: Sometimes I feel terrible after. I feel like just a terrible person with no patience and no ability to relate to people. That's just the worst.

CLINICIAN: What kind of impact has that had on your life day to day?

JEFF: Well, I'm all alone. It seems like women break up with me because they don't like my temper.

CLINICIAN: That's interesting. When you first came in for treatment, it was because you felt really sad and lonely. It sounds like the anger and depressed mood could be related. Thinking about it that way, does it make sense to you that we do some work on anger management?

JEFF: It seems okay.

In summary, clients can exhibit anger for many reasons. They might be testing the limits of the clinician, they might be scared or frustrated, and they might have had little experience communicating with others in a calmer and more rational way. Once clients see that the clinician is in control and can deal with their fear and frustration (even when they communicate in a calm tone), anger often abates. In cases in which it continues, clinicians should try to find some "hook" for some more focused work on anger management. By "hook," we mean a way to relate to the client's goals or presenting problems. Specifically, clinicians should help clients to identify the role that anger plays in their relationships outside of therapy (as was illustrated in the case of Jeff) and recognize ways that these relationships could improve if anger was less of a problem.

"My Client Is Overly Compliant"

In light of our earlier discussions on noncompliance, perhaps you might be wondering how clients could be *overly* compliant. Some clients agree with anything the clinician says, complete homework assignments flawlessly, and even push themselves beyond what the clinician suggests that they do. A client with OCD, for example, was sent home to spread contamination around her home. Her assignment was to allow her children to bring their backpacks in the house after school (she used to have the children leave them in the garage), to walk around the house wearing shoes she had worn outside, and to touch a small piece of fabric that she considered to be contaminated around uncontaminated things in the house like her favorite armchair and her bed. The client came in the following week having done all of these assignments—and more. One of her most feared activities was touching raw chicken or meat, for fear of getting ill or spreading contamination to her children. So, after rubbing her piece of contaminated fabric on her chair and bed and seeing that she could manage that, she took a piece of raw chicken and rubbed that on her chair and bed! This was an assignment that her clinician would have never suggested. It would be quite unpleasant (not to mention potentially unhealthy) to sit in a chair or sleep in a bed that had been doused in raw chicken juice. Although her clinician fully intended to tackle this concern with the client, he certainly would have come up with a more reasonable way of doing so—for example, having the client prepare chicken for dinner and then refraining from *excessively* washing her hands and kitchen utensils.

Solving the Problem

As with other behaviors, when clients are overly compliant in the context of therapy, we should use this as a clue to what life is like for them outside of therapy. This was very much the case with the client with OCD who went "beyond" her homework. At the time of treatment, the client was in a very difficult relationship. Despite all efforts, she was constantly criticized for being an incompetent wife and mother. Instead of leaving the relationship, she kept trying harder and harder to please. It seemed that she was applying these same efforts to her therapy— despite the fact that her clinician was certainly not being critical nor putting undue pressure on her to do the treatment "perfectly." A concern was that the motivation for doing the work of therapy was coming from her desire to please, instead of from intrinsic motivation to get over her OCD. This left her clinician feeling concerned that once therapy was over, the client would no longer make efforts to work on her OCD since her reinforcer for doing so (the clinician) would no longer be a presence in her life.

The clinician brought this up with the client. She agreed that she had been very concerned about doing the therapy correctly and was very worried that if she did not make enough effort, the clinician would get angry with her. The clinician corrected the client's misperceptions and was sure to more clearly set a supportive, noncritical tone in the therapeutic relationship. Furthermore, the clinician and client decided that it would be beneficial for the client to take a more active role in designing in-session exposures and homework assignments. By taking a more active role, the client felt that she had herself to answer to—not just the clinician.

A CONCLUSION: STAYING POSITIVE IN THE FACE OF CHALLENGES

If you are feeling pessimistic after reading this chapter, keep in mind that therapy typically runs quite smoothly. We all get a great deal of pleasure from working with pleasant clients who comply with treatment and who finish therapy with greatly improved functioning and quality of life.

This chapter has focused on cases that do not run quite so smoothly, but having such cases makes our work challenging and interesting. One of the special things about being a clinician is the feeling we get from helping clients move past obstacles that are preventing them from engaging in treatment and, in turn, making positive changes in their lives. We can all remember cases where, at some point in the therapy, we felt hopeless that the client would ever make the changes that he or she had set out to make. Figuring out what is standing in the client's way, and helping him or her to navigate past it, can be one of the most satisfying parts of our job. Whenever you are feeling frustrated, remember that human behavior is fascinating. Capitalize on your curiosity and use what you find out to help the client become a person who functions better in his or her world.

Chapter 10

■ ■ ■

TERMINATING THERAPY

In the previous chapters, we described the process of assessment and therapy and we considered how to manage various clinical difficulties that present themselves over the course of therapy. In this chapter, we discuss when and how to end therapy and highlight difficult clinical issues that can arise with respect to termination.

KEEPING THE END POINT IN MIND

CBT is a time-limited approach to treatment, and clients need to be made aware of this as soon as they begin therapy. Having a clear end point for the treatment process is beneficial in many ways. It provides clients with some external pressures to make changes by a specific time. Knowing that only four or five sessions remain often motivates clients to accomplish their most difficult goals. Believing that therapy can drag on indefinitely permits clients to move more slowly than they should.

Having an end point in mind also forces the clinician to constantly reevaluate the case conceptualization and whether the treatment plan is working. When therapy is time-limited, it cannot proceed aimlessly for a number of sessions. Rather, each session is structured and goal-oriented. Furthermore, each session must inform the subsequent session, in effect creating a path to termination. After each session, a clinician should ask him- or herself, "What do I need to do next to accomplish the goals of the therapy?"

In Michael's case, the primary goal of treatment was to help him with his social anxiety. The intention was to follow the protocol for so-

196

cial phobia that ran 16 sessions, including time at the end for goal setting and relapse prevention. However, there was flexibility in the plan
that would allow Michael and his clinician to address some of his other
problems. In Michael's case, the hierarchy of feared situations served as
a road map for the treatment. Cognitive restructuring techniques were
used to help Michael prepare for exposures and process what he had
learned from them once they were complete. Once an exposure was
done in session, a similar exposure was assigned for homework. If Michael came in for his next session still feeling that he needed to work on
that situation, another session could be dedicated to it. Otherwise, he
and his clinician would choose another situation to work on that was
further up the hierarchy. It was not essential that Michael conquer each
and every situation during the course of therapy. Rather, by the end of
therapy, it was intended that Michael have the skills to confront any situation on his own. In other words, the goal of treatment was to teach
Michael to be his own cognitive-behavioral therapist so he could continue to work on his social anxiety once treatment was over.

TEACHING CLIENTS TO BE THEIR OWN CLINICIANS

The idea of teaching clients to be their own therapists makes termination
more palatable to clients in CBT. Rather than framing termination as a
painful, frightening process, it is framed (from the very beginning of
therapy) as a very positive step. Terminating therapy means that clients
are ready to use their newly acquired skills to deal with their difficulties
on their own.

How can we ensure that clients are ready to be their own clinicians?
A key to accomplishing this goal is to gradually increase clients' involvement in the therapy process as it progresses. Clients must be encouraged
to take a gradually more active role in planning sessions and designing
homework. Early in therapy, the clinician will typically be quite directive
about the content of therapy sessions and about what the client should
do for homework. For example, Michael's clinician suggested that his
first exposure be a casual conversation; Michael and his clinician then
worked together to define the parameters of the exposure. After this exposure, the clinician assigned more casual conversations for homework,
helping Michael to identify upcoming events in the week in which opportunities for completing these exposures would exist. By being directive at this point in therapy, the clinician is essentially able to show the
client "the ropes." The client learns how to choose an exposure in a systematic way, how to define its parameters, carry it out, and then use it to
plan an appropriate homework exercise.

Later in treatment, it is essential that clients begin to make these decisions on their own. At the beginning of a session, they should play an active role in setting the agenda, and at the end of a session, they should design appropriate homework assignments. It is essential, particularly when clients are first taking on these roles, to be supportive. If they suggest a plan or design a homework assignment that seems unhelpful to you, do not be critical. Have them explain why they think the plan would be useful and, then, if you continue to have your doubts, try to guide the client in a graceful way to make appropriate adjustments. This should be done through Socratic questioning, rather than through the use of direct instructions.

Let's return to Michael's case to illustrate this point. As you recall, Michael's first exposure (in Session 5) was a casual conversation with a male stranger. For homework, Michael had lunch with some classmates and had to engage in casual conversation. When Michael came in for Session 6, he reported that he had a very good experience at the lunch but had been worrying a great deal about his blushing. He assumed that it was very noticeable, and he explained that "when people notice me blush, they assume that I am nervous and not so smart." In other words, completing the homework had brought up for Michael some very specific predictions about himself in social situations: (1) that people would notice him blushing, and (2) that people would assume that this physical symptom meant that he was not smart. As a result, in Session 6, Michael had another conversation with a male stranger (a replication of the exposure from Session 5) but used the exposure to evaluate some different predictions that he did not explore in the previous session. This exposure was also very beneficial for Michael—the individual with whom he chatted did not notice his blushing at all, and when asked what he thought of people who do blush, he reported, "They are just built that way. Some people blush more than others. It doesn't mean anything." Michael found this feedback very helpful, and when he met his same friends for lunch in the week following Session 6, he reported feeling far less concerned with blushing.

In Session 7, Michael's clinician asked him to look at his hierarchy and suggest an exposure for them to work on:

CLINICIAN: Michael, what would you like to do in today's session?

MICHAEL: I'd like to have another casual conversation. Doing that over these past 2 weeks has been really helpful.

CLINICIAN: Great. You also had some casual conversations for homework too, didn't you?

MICHAEL: Yeah. They went really well. I really saw that I was able to carry on a good conversation over lunch with my friends, and since last week I am worrying a lot less about blushing.

CLINICIAN: That's great. Do you think it would be helpful to do more casual conversations today? Or, would it be helpful to move on to something else?

MICHAEL: Hmmm. I guess I was feeling so good about the conversations, I wanted to do more. But, now that I think about it, it probably is a good idea to move on.

CLINICIAN: Why is that?

MICHAEL: Well, I feel pretty good about conversations now and know that I am not going to avoid them anymore out there in the "real world." I really grabbed lots of opportunities last week and I know that I am going to keep doing that this week. So, knowing that I am not avoiding and that I feel pretty good about things, it seems like we should tackle something a bit higher up on my hierarchy.

CLINICIAN: I think that is an excellent plan, Michael. What are you thinking of?

MICHAEL: Well, I haven't tackled all conversations! I am feeling pretty good chatting with guys now, but chatting with women is much harder for me. Do you think I should start working on that?

CLINICIAN: I think that's an excellent plan. Let's put "casual conversation with a woman" on our agenda for today.

By not simply correcting Michael, the clinician forced him to be his own therapist and think through different options for the session. In doing so, Michael realized that he had accomplished one aspect of casual conversations (with male peers) which infused the session with a positive tone and helped him to draw on this sense of confidence for the next item on his hierarchy (conversing with female peers).

Another really useful tool in helping clients to be their own therapists is to have them play the role of therapist. There are a few ways to do this. When clients tell you about something that was problematic for them or that they fear will be problematic for them, you can say, "If you were a therapist, what would you suggest?" One caveat is not to employ this line of questioning too early in therapy. It can be intimidating for clients to be put on the spot this way, and they might wonder why they are coming for therapy at all if the clinician refuses to tell them how to do anything. When your rapport with the client is stronger, however, and when you feel confident that clients know how to respond to the question, this technique can be very effective. Clients see that they can help themselves in much the same way as you help them. Another way to have clients "be the therapist" is to do a role play in which the therapist takes on the role of client. Clients then have to instruct this mock client on how to solve a problem. Finally, particularly near the end of therapy, the clinician can provide the client with some scenarios of difficult situations that may come up once treatment is over and ask the client how he or she would manage them.

Another excellent way to make sure that clients are ready to be their own clinicians is to look for evidence of these abilities and reinforce them. This evidence is most salient when situations arise in clients' lives just by chance (i.e., that were not assigned for homework) and the client deals with these events effectively using CBT techniques. Consider the following example from a session with a client who presented for treatment of depression:

CLIENT: I had a few rough spots this week. Kind of made me nervous since we're so near the end of treatment.

CLINICIAN: Why don't you tell me about them?

CLIENT: It kind of got going at work on Monday. I had given a letter to my boss to read over and he gave it back to me with red edits everywhere. It looked just awful.

CLINICIAN: What did you think when you got the letter back?

CLIENT: At first, I thought I had totally screwed up. I felt really down. I just sat there for a few minutes feeling bad, feeling like a total failure.

CLINICIAN: And then?

CLIENT: Then I snapped out of it. I really thought it through. This was a really important letter that my boss had told me repeatedly that we had to get "just right." It's funny because once I thought it through, I realized that we had talked a lot about how important it was, but we never actually reviewed what we wanted to say. So I had a go at it and I guess what I had done didn't quite map onto what my boss wanted.

CLINICIAN: And?

CLIENT: Well, then I didn't feel so bad. My boss had been thinking about this a lot and he clearly had a vision of what this letter was going to say. I can see why he then went through and changed a lot of what I did. It had nothing to do with me, really.

CLINICIAN: So you fixed the letter?

CLIENT: I did. And, I took it back to Bob's office. He looked up from what he was doing and apologized for all that red on my original letter. He told me that he had kind of drafted a letter in his mind and should have just written it himself. He said that mine was great but that he got stuck on the way of doing it that he had come up with over the weekend.

CLINICIAN: It sounds like you were really able to step back and think through some of those initial automatic thoughts you had. That's really wonderful. How do you feel about it?

CLIENT: I feel great. A few months ago this would have sent me to the bathroom in tears and then for days I'd feel down. This week, it was about 5 minutes of feeling bad and then I got out of it. I was really happy.

One final point deserves emphasis with respect to clients learning to be their own therapists. Many clinicians, particularly those who are beginners, forget to positively reinforce clients for such efforts. When clients seize an opportunity in their lives to try out what they have learned or come to a very useful insight during a session, we should praise them. This is not to suggest that we should go over the top with praise for our clients. Rather, when they do something that we know will serve them well, let them know it, and do so with enthusiasm. The positive feedback from the clinician and most importantly, the positive reinforcement gained in the natural environment both instill hope in clients that they are capable of making positive changes in their lives.

THINGS TO DO IN THE LAST FEW SESSIONS OF THERAPY

When both clinician and client feel confident that the client knows how to be his or her own therapist, the time has probably come to terminate therapy. However, there are some important topics to cover before finishing: The client needs to have a clear sense of what he or she has accomplished; the client needs to set some goals for the future; the clinician must ensure that the client has realistic expectations for the future; and the client must know what to do if symptoms reemerge.

Helping Clients See What They Have Accomplished in Treatment

As treatment progresses and clients begin to function better, they often forget where they were when they started treatment. Helping clients to see how much progress they have made is very important. Keep in mind that when termination comes up, some clients worry that they have not changed enough and therefore need to stay in therapy until they are "perfect." Perfection is, of course, an impossible goal to attain. Showing clients how far they have come, despite being left with some difficulties, can make them feel more ready to terminate treatment. Furthermore, if clients have gradually taken a more active role in the therapy, clinicians can help them to see the role that they played in their improvement and the role that they will continue to play on their own (e.g., serving as their own therapist).

How can you help clients to see the improvements that they have made? An excellent way to accomplish this is to compare measures from the initial assessment with how the client is currently doing. In most settings, an in-depth clinical interview will not be performed at the end of treatment. Nevertheless, interviewing techniques can be used to help clients recognize change. If a structured clinical interview was originally used, it can be useful to spend some time with clients assessing whether criteria are still met for a particular disorder. Regardless of whether the initial evaluation was carried out using a structured or unstructured interview format, it can be extremely useful to spend some time with clients discussing their quality of life and how it has changed since the beginning of treatment. If a client began therapy barely being able to get out of bed and ended therapy working part-time and spending more time with her children, this would be an excellent way to articulate progress.

In Chapter 3, we discussed a number of other tools for assessment in addition to interviews. These, too, can be useful in helping clients to see the degree to which they have changed over the course of therapy. We discussed using observational techniques to see, for example, how close to a feared stimulus a client could get. The behavior test can be re-administered at the end of treatment to measure change. Following the example of a specific phobia of spiders, it can be remarkable for a client to be able to hold a spider in his hand at the end of treatment when at the beginning he could only be in the room with a spider if it was in a sealed jar.

Self-monitoring can be used in much the same way. When discussing self-monitoring, we brought up the case of a 16-year-old with trichotillomania. During the assessment, the client was asked to keep track of how many hairs she pulled each day. Once she started treatment, she continued to monitor her pulling, and each week, she and her clinician would plot these data in a graph. It was remarkable for the client to see the decrease in pulling from week to week, and, even more so, to see that she had gone from pulling hundreds of hairs per day to pulling none at all by the end of treatment.

If a hierarchy of feared situations was created during therapy, it can be helpful to re-rate the hierarchy at the end of treatment. Clients like to see how much less discomfort they experience in response to these situations and feel very good when situations that were previously problematic are no longer a concern.

Finally, questionnaires can also be used to demonstrate change to clients. Though we do not want to provide clients with raw scores from measures (since these will not be meaningful to them), clients often like to hear the degree to which they have changed over the course of treatment. For example, clients can be told that they have reported an 80% reduction in their symptoms since first coming in for treatment.

Some clients do not make the kinds of changes that they (and their clinicians) had hoped they would make in treatment. With these clients, discussing progress is more difficult. It is most often the case that clients make *some* change in therapy. In this light, it can still be useful to discuss progress—even it was minimal—and then to give some thought to what the client can do to make further progress.

Many clients who do not do well in therapy were resistant to some aspect of the treatment. For example, a client might refuse to do any cognitive restructuring on her own in between sessions. Such clients leave a therapy session feeling quite good, but without doing any work on their difficulties during the week, they come back the following week back to where they started. Similarly, some clients refuse to do certain behavioral exercises that their clinicians see as crucial to the treatment process.

It is important in such cases to help clients to see why treatment did not go as well as had been hoped. It is crucial here to be sensitive to clients—typically, when clients do not do the work that they should be doing in therapy, it is not because they are lazy or trying to be argumentative with the clinician. Rather, sometimes clients come to therapy before they are ready to do the work that they need to do to make significant changes in their lives. Throughout treatment, we tell clients what they need to do to make these changes. Therefore, it will come as no surprise if we reiterate these "requirements," helping clients to see that when they are ready to more fully engage in the therapy, it is likely that they will be able to make the changes that they desire.

Helping Clients to Set Goals for the Future

Ending therapy can be daunting for some clients because they do not feel as if they are completely "done" working on their difficulties. Once weekly contact with the clinician is over, they worry that they will no longer know what to do or how to do it.

A good way to alleviate these concerns is to work with clients in the last few sessions of therapy to set future goals. These goals should be aimed at helping clients to maintain and expand the gains made in treatment. It is good to assign a timeline for accomplishing the goals (e.g., within the next 2 weeks, I want to invite two friends to coffee or to a movie; within a month, I want to get the projects done around the house that I have been putting off; within 3 months, I'd like to have a new job) and to make sure the timeline is realistic (e.g., getting a new job in 3 months is realistic, getting a new job next week might not be). Beyond simply listing goals (e.g., I want to get a job), the clinician and client should consider how each goal will be accomplished and whether there are smaller goals to attain along the way. In seeking out a new job, the client might want to meet with a job counselor, do some mock interviews, work on his résumé, and speak to some people who already work in his field of interest, for example. Clinicians and their clients should also consider, and work through, potential roadblocks to accomplishing these goals.

Establishing Realistic Expectations for the Future

As clients near the end of therapy, we also need to examine the expectations that they hold for the future once therapy is over. Many clients come to therapy expecting that they will never encounter problems again in the future. In some cases, clients really do leave therapy no longer having the difficulties for which they sought help. In other cases, clients leave with some continuing difficulties or residual symptoms—things they still need to deal with and perhaps will always need to deal with. It is important to discuss expectations with clients early in therapy. CBT is premised on giving people skills to deal with difficulties as they arise. Thus, while the goal of therapy is certainly a reduction in distress and an improvement in functioning, perhaps the overarching goal is acquisition of new skills that will help clients continue to deal with residual difficulties after therapy, as well as new difficulties that might arise in the future.

Discussing with Clients What to Do If Symptoms Reemerge

It is important that our clients know that termination of therapy does not mean they need to manage on their own forever. Difficulties do reemerge, and sometimes clients forget what they have learned in CBT or begin to have difficulties applying what they have learned. At these times, a few booster sessions, or even another course of therapy, might be needed.

This brings us back to the importance of realistic expectations. For people who have had psychological difficulties once, it is quite likely that at some point they might have some difficulties again. A client who was treated for an eating disorder might begin to have new concerns about shape and weight after becoming pregnant. Similarly, a client who completed treatment for alcohol dependence might become concerned around holiday time when he knows that he will be in many situations where alcohol is being served.

The best way to ensure that these "bumps in the road" will not quickly progress to full-blown relapse is to prepare clients for their occurrence and to normalize them. All clients should be taught to expect such bumps along the way. If they do not expect them, experiencing them can be very troubling. Clients might see themselves as failures— "I'm losing everything that I learned," or "This is just another thing I've totally failed at." This state of negativity can indeed lead people to engage in dysfunctional behaviors. For example, the pregnant client might binge to escape her negative feelings about herself.

Clients must understand before completing treatment that lapses tend to occur before full-blown relapse. There is a lot that clients can do to prevent the progression to a complete return of difficulties. First, they need to understand that these lapses signal an opportunity to practice the skills that they learned in therapy. A nice thing to do with clients before termination is to make a summary sheet of what they have learned in therapy and what techniques were helpful to them. This might include a list of rational responses to counter automatic thoughts (e.g., "People judge me for the kind of person I am, not for my weight") and some thoughts on how to refrain from engaging in dysfunctional behaviors (e.g., eat three normal meals and two snacks a day; when the urge to binge comes on, call a friend, take a walk, or do something else distracting to see if the urge will pass; etc.). When clients are having a difficult time, they can refer back to this sheet and remember what they found useful during CBT.

Clients should also know when it is appropriate to call their clinician. Again, the progression from a lapse to full-blown relapse does not happen overnight. Clients should be encouraged not to wait until relapse occurs to contact their clinician. They might feel silly calling about minimal problems (e.g., a few days of dysfunctional thinking, a few urges to engage in an unhealthy behavior, etc.), but if they know in advance that doing so is fine, they will do it. Clinicians can assess the situation and then decide how to proceed. Sometimes, a supportive phone call and some advice on applying what they have learned in therapy will do clients a world of good. At other times, the clinician might suggest a few "booster" sessions to help clients get back to where they were before the lapse.

In summary, there are a few things we should be doing and looking out for before terminating therapy with clients. First and foremost, we want to ensure that clients understand the core CBT techniques and know how to use them. As we have said, clients need to know how to be their own therapists. We also want to help clients set goals for what they would like to accomplish once therapy is over. Few clients feel "perfect" at the end of treatment, and most appreciate taking some time to consider what they would like to continue working on and how to apply the skills that they have learned in therapy to these goals.

We want to strike a balance between helping clients see all the progress that they have made in therapy and maintaining a realistic mindset about what the future might hold. Even if they still have some difficulties, it does not mean therapy was a failure. Similarly, they should expect that difficulties of some kind or another might arise again in the future. Again, this does not make the client a failure—encountering difficulties on the road of life is part of the human experience. What clients need to know is that they have the skills to deal with these bumps along the road.

TERMINATING THERAPY: STAYING THE COURSE OR MAKING ADJUSTMENTS?

We now know what needs to be done before the end of therapy, but we are left with the question of when exactly that end should come. As we have noted, cognitive-behavioral clinicians make a prediction of how long therapy is likely to last when they first start seeing a client. Most of the time, the predictions are reasonably accurate and therapy proceeds for the predicted length of time. For various reasons, however, therapy sometimes ends sooner or later than expected.

Early Termination

Terminating Early for "Good Reason"

When we think about premature termination of therapy, we tend to frame it in a negative light. Therapy is terminated early for clients who are noncompliant or who drop out of treatment before we think that they should. Sometimes, however, therapy is terminated early because clients make faster gains than expected. When clients are presented with the CBT rationale, some just "get it" very quickly. Even before we begin active interventions in therapy, they begin to apply the concepts and see improvements. These clients may not need a full course of therapy. As we already mentioned, the overarching goals of CBT are to teach clients skills and to help them learn how to apply these skills. Some clients accomplish these goals more quickly than others and begin quite rapidly to see positive changes in their lives.

It can sometimes be anxiety provoking to discontinue treatment with a client after a relatively short course. While the clinician and client might be very happy with the gains, they might worry about how easily they came. A good solution to these concerns is to extend the time between sessions rather than discontinuing completely. For clients who were coming for weekly sessions, biweekly sessions can be instituted for a few weeks. Similarly, if clients stop coming to sessions, weekly phone calls can be set for the first few weeks posttermination to check that clients are maintaining their gains.

When the Clinician Decides to Terminate Treatment Early

Despite the clinician's best efforts to motivate clients and get them involved in treatment, some simply refuse to do so. Perhaps one of the most difficult things to learn about doing therapy is figuring out when it is time to stop persevering with unresponsive clients and discontinue treatment. For people who have become clinicians because they want to help people, "firing" a client from treatment can be a very wrenching experience. Particularly for beginning clinicians, dismissing clients from therapy can have all sorts of negative connotations. Clinicians often personalize the situation, believing that if they were more skilled, things would have turned out differently. Beginning clinicians can also find it difficult to face the fact that people are not always able or willing to help themselves. There is no magic way to know whether or not to discontinue treatment. In our experience, a good way is to focus on concrete indices. On the simplest level, the important question to ask yourself is "Is the client *willingly engaged* in the treatment?" If sessions are spent *convincing* clients of the rationale for CBT, or discussing why homework was not completed, or arguing about what should happen in the session that day, the client is not engaged in the treatment. Sometimes, the situation is not so clear because clients will do *some* work, but it will not come without struggle. In other words, you will sense that the client is not doing the treatment in an optimal way.

When clients are not engaged in the treatment, CBT cannot work. By keeping clients in therapy, we are setting them up for failure, with two potentially negative results. First, clients will finish treatment feeling bad about themselves. They will have come to sessions for several weeks or months and made virtually no changes in their lives. Second, clients will leave treatment with a negative view of CBT. They will come to view it as a treatment that does not work, or perhaps as a treatment that will not work for them. This bodes poorly for the future—if clients do get to a point where they are more motivated to work on their difficulties, their motivation might be sapped by a belief that the treatment will not work anyway.

In a sense then, dismissing clients from therapy does them a favor. Rather than framing it as a punishment ("I won't work with you anymore because you're not doing what I am asking you to do"), terminating therapy early can be viewed as a temporary decision. The clinician and client should discuss how it is not a good time right now for the client to be in therapy, but that he or she should feel free to come back and try again when truly ready to engage in the treatment. Undoubtedly, it is better for clients to come back and try therapy when they are ready and to then succeed, than to sit through a course of therapy when they are not ready and to fail.

When the Client Decides to Terminate Treatment Early

Sometimes the decision to terminate treatment early comes from clients. This can be problematic when clients' decisions to discontinue treatment do not mesh with the sense that the clinician has of the case. Clearly, we cannot force people to continue in therapy when they do not want to. However, before simply accepting clients' decisions, it is important to explore why they want to leave.

Clients choose to discontinue therapy for a number of reasons, but a very common reason is that they believe that it is not working. This is an issue that must be addressed since clients' expectancies play a role in treatment outcome. Therapy can "not work" for a whole host of reasons. First, therapy can take some time to work. Immediate results should not be expected. Clients need to learn CBT skills, apply them, and then give themselves time to have experiences that change their beliefs about given situations. On a related note, therapy is not going to solve all of a client's difficulties. Clinicians can help clients to maintain a hopeful outlook by setting reasonable goals and delineating the steps that they need to take to accomplish these goals.

Some clients prematurely discontinue therapy because they are not willing to do the required work. As we already discussed, it is important to realize that some clients are simply not ready to change when they come for treatment. Some clients are forced to come to therapy by spouses, parents, family members, or friends. When motivation does not come from within, clients have a much harder time engaging in therapy. Even when clients come on their own accord, problems can arise. If the perceived benefits of doing the treatment do not outweigh the costs (e.g., having to make time for therapy, making difficult changes), clients will also have difficulty engaging. It is hard as a clinician to think that clients' lives sometimes need to become *more* difficult before they are ready to truly engage in treatment, but it is absolutely true. It is often best to go along with clients' decisions and invite them to come back for treatment when they feel more ready. They will be more likely to succeed at such a time, and your work together will progress much more smoothly.

Before moving on, it is important to address the reactions that beginning clinicians can have to clients prematurely terminating therapy. This can be a difficult situation to cope with at first. As we have already pointed out, beginning clinicians often believe that if they were more experienced, the client would have engaged in the therapy and would have made significant improvements in his or her life. To some extent, this might be true. More seasoned clinicians are more accustomed to dealing with client noncompliance and might be better able to motivate clients. However, clinician experience does not explain all the variance in these situations—while we most certainly need to do our part in motivating clients and instilling confidence in the treatment, clients also need to come to therapy ready and willing to do the hard work. A difficult thing to learn as a beginning clinician is that we cannot help everyone who comes through the door. An easier way to come to terms with this realization is to know that we cannot help everyone *at the time* they walk through our door. It is a job well done when we can encourage a noncompliant client to come back for therapy when he or she is ready. When this is done in a positive, noncritical way, it is quite possible that clients will come back and will succeed when they do.

Extending Therapy

When the Clinician Decides to Extend Treatment

Case conceptualization involves an ongoing evaluation of how the therapy is progressing. Sometimes new difficulties come up that were not considered in the original conceptualization of the case. Some additional time might need to be allotted to dealing with these issues. Similarly, some clients do not improve at the rate that we would have expected. We have all had experiences with clients who really start to "get it" and make significant improvements close to the end of treatment. This kind of client might catch on a little later than other clients, but it would be a shame to discontinue treatment just because an end date has arrived. A few extra sessions of treatment might be indicated. Making this kind of adjustment does not mean extending therapy indefinitely. Rather, the original plan for the treatment is revisited and adjustments to it are clearly articulated. For example, the clinician might suggest adding five extra sessions for the client who caught on to the treatment techniques quite near to the originally agreed-upon end of treatment.

When the Client Wants to Extend Treatment

Sometimes it is the client who does not want to end treatment. Some clients will be direct and simply say they are not ready to terminate. Others will be more subtle, suddenly bringing up new problems just as a very successful course of treatment is coming to an end or start to miss sessions when they used to be very diligent about coming.

Why might clients begin to engage in these behaviors? The most likely possibility is that clients are hesitant about making a go of it on their own. It may be hard for them to imagine maintaining their gains without weekly reassurance from their clinician. These concerns can be dealt with by coming back to the CBT rationale about clients learning to be their own therapists. Clients can be reassured that they do have the skills to manage on their own. Furthermore, arrangements can be put in place so that therapy is tapered gradually. Rather than extending the number of sessions, the last few sessions can be held every other week instead of every week, giving clients the opportunity to try managing on their own while still having the reassurance of periodically checking in with the clinician. Some clients see the end of regularly scheduled visits as the absolute end of contact with the clinician. It can also be very reassuring to clients to simply tell them that they can call or come in once in a while to check in (particularly if they begin to encounter problems again).

Another possible explanation for why clients do not want to terminate is that the therapeutic relationship might be one of the only positive parts of their lives. Letting go of something so reinforcing can be difficult and, as mentioned earlier, clients might report new symptoms or keep missing the "last session" to prolong the inevitability of parting. These feelings are important to deal with, and that might mean extending the therapy. On the one hand, you are reinforcing the client's avoidance of termination. On the other, if a specific agreement can be made of how long the therapy will be extended and what issues will be discussed, a few additional sessions can be beneficial to the client. Rather than veering off into treating new problems, a better use of time would be to deal directly with separation issues and help clients begin to forge some meaningful social relationships outside of therapy.

A RETURN TO THE CASE OF MICHAEL

As you will recall, Michael's treatment was slated to last between 16 and 20 sessions. The plan was to focus on treatment for social phobia, dealing with other related problems as they came up. Michael's treatment progressed "by the book" until about Session 10. He was very compliant with treatment, easy to get along with, and made gains even quicker than would have been predicted. In terms of the case conceptualization, it began to seem as if Michael's uncertainties about his career were greatly explained by social anxiety. As he began to feel more comfortable in his various roles (student, clergy, etc.), he also began to feel more and more confident that the priesthood was a good path for him. As we noted in the previous chapter, Michael also started to believe that his family was more "on board" with his choices and that any reservations that they continued to have were more their issues than his. The topic of Michael having his own family did not come up during this part of therapy, and his clinician did not push the issue since it was not one that Michael came into therapy wanting to discuss. Michael spoke about these issues from time to time with his mentors at the seminary, and it was quite clear to his clinician that he felt more comfortable discussing these issues with them than with her.

Given Michael's excellent progress, at Session 10, his clinician suggested to him that they terminate therapy before the agreed-upon 16 to 20 sessions. Michael seemed very happy with this suggestion and felt that he now possessed the skills to be his own therapist. It was agreed that two more sessions would be dedicated to specific exposures that Michael still wanted to work on and to beginning to discuss relapse prevention and goal setting. One final session would serve as a "wrap-up" session to finish discussing relapse prevention and goal setting and to help Michael reflect on all the progress he had made.

When Michael came in for Session 11, the clinical picture shifted. For the first time since treatment began, Michael refused to do an exposure. He and his therapist had planned for him to do an unrehearsed sermon, arguably an item at the top of his hierarchy, but even so, this refusal was very out of character for Michael. He then started to tell his clinician that he was not ready to discontinue therapy and that he felt he needed at least 20 sessions in total, if not more.

Michael's clinician took this at face value at first. She assumed that his anxiety about the planned exposure took him aback and made him wonder if he was indeed prepared to be his own therapist. Could he handle stressful situations as they came up, once he was no longer coming to weekly therapy sessions? She started to ask Michael what he could have done before coming in for the session to feel more confident about doing the exposure. Michael responded in exactly the way his clinician would have hoped—he could have done some cognitive restructuring and come up with a helpful rational response, he could have reminded himself of how well the other exposures had gone which also seemed daunting at first, and he certainly could have called the clinician to discuss modifying the planned exposure to be slightly less difficult. Michael was able to provide all of these possible solutions, but did not seem to have used them when he needed them. His clinician then switched gears and asked whether anything notable had happened during the week. At this point, Michael revealed that something very notable had indeed happened.

Two weeks before, Michael received a phone call from the sister of a close childhood friend of his. Sarah was coming into town for some meetings for work and asked if Michael could show her around and join her for a few dinners. Michael felt some anxiety about getting together with her, but decided to visit with her anyway. He had known Sarah when they were children and thought it would be nice to catch up with her, and, furthermore, he viewed it as yet another opportunity to work on his social anxiety. What Michael had not expected was that he would have feelings for her.

Since the last session, Michael had taken Sarah around the city for a day of sightseeing and had met her for dinner every night. He was captivated by her warmth and gregariousness, and he found himself feeling very attracted to her physically as well. He could not remember the last time he had so enjoyed himself. While he was slightly anxious, he was amazed by how little of a role social anxiety played in their interaction. Early in their week together, Sarah had joked about it being "too bad" that he was going to be a priest, but the previous night she had come right out and asked him how set on this path he was. Michael, who was so certain of his path just one week before, all of a sudden did not know how to answer this question.

When Michael shared this story with his clinician, she began by validating his feelings and thanking him for sharing it with her. He explained that she was the only person he could speak to about this. Speaking to his superiors at the seminary was out of the question, and he felt that speaking to his family would unfairly stir up their hopes that Michael might still make the decision to return to his career in medicine, marry, and have a family of his own. For now, his clinician accepted this, but made a mental note that his hesitation fit very well with Michael's concerns about making mistakes and suffering rejection. Michael seemed very reluctant to share with people that he might be having second thoughts.

Michael's clinician then shared with him a revised conceptualization of his case. In effect, what he was encountering was a double-edged sword, of sorts. As his social anxiety improved, he felt more certain that he could enter the priesthood, do well at it, and enjoy it. Yet, with the improvement in social anxiety, Michael was also able to put himself in a position to consider having a romantic relationship—also something he could now "do well at" and enjoy. Successful treatment for social anxiety opened doors for him, but also introduced complications. Michael related to this conceptualization, and at the end of the session he admitted that he would have been fine to do the planned exposure for the day. He just did not want to do it, because suddenly it did not seem terribly important. When his clinician asked why he chose not to recount the story of Sarah right away, rather than trying to dodge the exposure, Michael explained that he was not sure when he came into the session whether he was going to share it or not. He felt that by sharing it he was opening up the real possibility that the priesthood might not be right for him. After coming to feel sure that it was, this new doubt was quite daunting.

At the end of the session, Michael and his clinician agreed to "shift gears" and spend a few weeks discussing the conflict between wanting a wife and family but also wanting to enter the priesthood. They did not establish a set number of sessions, but rather decided to see how things proceeded week to week. Michael and his clinician spent three more sessions together after this one. During this time, Michael remained in touch with Sarah and continued to have positive feelings toward her. At the same time, she lived far away and it seemed unlikely that they would ever establish a relationship. However, Michael and his clinician were able to view Sarah as a symbol of what Michael would give up, if he were to become a priest.

During these three remaining sessions, the initial underlying mechanism for Michael's problems—concerns about making mistakes and being rejected—remained very much a part of treatment. Michael's clinician thought that he might benefit at this time from the support of his superiors at work and his family and recognized that his reluctance to speak to them was spurred by the belief that they would think he had made a terrible mistake in deciding to try out the priesthood for a year and would give up on him. Cognitive restructuring was used to help Michael challenge this belief. He came to recognize that this special "trial" year must exist for this very reason—providing people the time to carefully think through this major life decision. He looked at some literature he had from the church reporting the percentage of people who entered this trial year and then did not join the priesthood. These data showed him that many people do "change their minds." He also recognized that changing his mind was unlikely to cause much upset in his family (in fact, he believed they would be pleased), and although it might cause some upset in the church, he felt that ultimately they too would forgive him.

This process of cognitive restructuring led Michael to seek advice from his family and a trusted clergy person. Both felt great empathy for the struggle he was going through and both offered unique insights that

Michael would not have received had he only spoken with his clinician. Michael did not see any evidence to support his belief that he would be judged negatively for "making a mistake," nor that he would be rejected. He came to see that he had not, in fact, made a mistake, but rather was reconsidering a decision that was crucially important to both his career and personal life.

An interesting "twist" on Michael's case was the "involvement" of God. Michael felt that he had experienced a calling from God to become a priest and that he would be looked on with displeasure if he did not answer this calling. In working on these beliefs, Michael considered behavioral changes that he could make if he indeed returned to secular life. He considered becoming a lay pastor at a local hospital, as well as volunteering at some programs for underprivileged children at his local church. Now that social anxiety was less of a problem, Michael was able to consider all sorts of ways that he might be able to serve God.

The core concern about making mistakes and being rejected also arose when Michael and his clinician discussed interactions with women. If Michael did leave the priesthood, the expectation would then be that he would start dating and eventually meet someone to marry. Given that this was not an area worked on in treatment (all of his casual conversations with women were with clinic staff, nuns, or parishioners), Michael was concerned that he would not be able to manage it. He feared that he would "mess up" every date and ruin all of his chances, leaving him alone and unhappy.

In response to these concerns, Michael's clinician helped him to appreciate how much he had enjoyed meeting Sarah and also helped him to see how the skills he had learned in therapy would apply to dating, just as they had applied to a range of other social situations. They discussed what it meant to "mess up" a date, appreciated that he would likely mess up some (as all people do!), but that this did not mean a lifetime of loneliness. Michael's clinician also reassured him that if dating was very problematic for him, they could work on it in some additional sessions of therapy. Although he seemed to be leaning in the direction of leaving the priesthood, Michael's clinician never pressured him to make a decision, appreciating that the process might take some time

These discussions occurred during the three sessions of therapy after Michael met Sarah. At this point, a firm decision had not been made about Michael's future. Following the third session, the clinician received a phone message from Michael. He had left the seminary, was on his way back to his hometown, and did not know what his next step would be. All he knew was that the priesthood was not for him. He left no forwarding information.

The abruptness of Michael's decision took his clinician aback. She was disappointed that they would not have the opportunity to continue on this journey together. It seemed, however, that Michael had made his decision and that it was painful for him. He had moved to the town only because the seminary was located there. It made sense to his clinician that he would return to his former town, where he owned a home, had some friends and work colleagues, and had a job that he could come back to at any time. It was likely that Michael would bring his newly ac-quired skills home with him and use them to get the support that he needed.

Chapter 11

■ ■ ■

THE PROCESS OF SUPERVISION

In this book, we have followed the course of CBT from initial contact with clients, to assessment, to treatment, and to termination. We have also discussed how to deal with challenges that arise during this process. Our intention is to help beginning clinicians navigate their way through this process without undue anxiety. In addition to acquiring knowledge and clinical experience, beginning clinicians have another tool to help them with this process—their supervisors.

In this chapter, we frame the process of supervision in much the same way as we have framed the process of therapy. Supervision is vital for acquiring the skills of case conceptualization, differential diagnosis, treatment planning, and implementation. However, the process of supervision does not come without its own set of difficulties, sometimes about these very training issues. Furthermore, difficulties of a more interpersonal nature can also arise in the supervisory relationship. In this chapter, we offer advice on how best to resolve these issues so that the goals of supervision can be accomplished.

THE GOALS OF SUPERVISION

One of the ultimate goals of a graduate education in the mental health professions is to prepare students to competently deliver treatment services to individuals who are experiencing psychological difficulties. The first step in this process is training through coursework. However, no classroom instruction can completely prepare a student for the experience of being with a client and, therefore, classroom instruction is usually followed by practical experience in which students develop their clinical skills. Because developing clinicians are not yet self-sufficient and independently competent, they require monitoring by a clinical supervisor whose job is to provide support and feedback during the training process.

From a didactic perspective, the goal of supervision is to teach the skills required to offer psychological services. From a more pragmatic perspective, it is also important that students obtain the training that they need for completion of their training program and licensure. Students are responsible for ensuring that they obtain the amount of training (e.g., number of hours engaged in direct clinical activities, number of hours of supervision) and the type of training that they will need for licensure. The qualifications of the supervisor will also be considered and, in most jurisdictions, clinical hours only "count" toward licensure if they have been supervised by a licensed psychologist. Trainees in other fields (e.g., psychiatry, social work, psychiatric nursing, etc.) should learn about the guidelines for licensure in their respective areas.

THE ROLES OF THE SUPERVISOR

Before discussing how the process of supervision works, it is interesting to consider the roles of the supervisor and the trainee within the supervisory relationship. Clinical supervisors perform three main functions— they train beginning clinicians, they ensure that clients receive competent care, and, in many cases, they also serve a mentorship role.

Training Beginning Therapists

The training function of clinical supervisors is to help trainees hone their assessment, case conceptualization, treatment planning, and implementation skills. Typically, these skills are taught according to the supervisor's orientation—trainees learn to think about psychological difficulties and how to treat them from a specific framework (such as the cognitive-behavioral framework).

In addition to being taught how to *do* assessments and therapy, supervisors teach trainees about *being* clinicians. They help trainees learn how to deal with difficult issues that can arise in therapy. They also teach beginning clinicians how to practice psychology in an ethical and moral manner by introducing to them the ethical codes that govern our work and helping them to resolve ethical dilemmas as they arise.

Invariably, in the context of this training, supervisors are also required to evaluate the performance of their trainees. When people think of an "evaluation," they often think of a final assessment of work at the time when a supervisory relationship is ending. Although this final evaluation is undoubtedly important, evaluation is probably best thought of as an ongoing process over the duration of the supervisory relationship, much like case conceptualization with clients over the course of the therapeutic relationship. It would be very unhelpful for students to be evaluated only when a supervisory relationship is ending. Rather, evaluation should be an iterative process where feedback at each meeting will then influence subsequent work until the next supervision meeting.

Ensuring Competent Care

Perhaps the most important role of the supervisor is to ensure the welfare of clients. In fact, supervisors are legally and ethically liable for any harm done by a trainee under their supervision. Thus, supervisors must always be aware of the status, treatment course, and current level of functioning of each client. Obviously, it is the trainee's responsibility to share this information, but it is the supervisor's responsibility to be available to listen to it and to offer feedback and guidance.

Mentoring

Many clinical supervisors, in addition to teaching clients how to do therapy, serve as mentors for their trainees. Mentorship may involve helping trainees to decide what kind of supervisory experiences they would like to gain once the current experience has been completed. It might also involve helping trainees to chart their career paths. Perhaps the aspect of mentoring that is most often overlooked is helping trainees gain skills that will allow them to serve as supervisors in the future. Supervisors can discuss with their trainees their own personal style of supervision and how it has developed over the course of their career. Furthermore, some supervisors will permit senior trainees to supervise more junior trainees. The supervisor will then provide feedback on supervision skills to the more advanced student. This kind of experience is a very valuable one and should be taken advantage of, if available.

THE ROLE OF THE TRAINEE

The major role of the trainee is to provide clinical services to individuals who have sought help for psychological difficulties. The expectation, of course, is that trainees will provide the best services that they possibly can. How can this be accomplished? First, as we discussed earlier in the book, beginning clinicians must do everything that they can to prepare for their work with clients. Second, clinicians must be knowledgeable about ethical and legal standards and must uphold them in all of their dealings with clients. They must also be aware of personal issues and how these might negatively affect their work. Finally, most relevant to this chapter, trainees must make good use of supervision. As we discuss in greater detail later in the chapter, this means setting up supervision meetings, coming to meetings well prepared, being open to feedback, making changes wherever necessary, and knowing conditions under which to seek supervision outside of regularly scheduled meetings.

SETTING UP A SUPERVISORY RELATIONSHIP

Choosing a Supervisor

Over the course of your training, there will be varying degrees of choice in who serves as your supervisor. In some situations, you will be assigned to a supervisor in a particular setting. In other situations, you may choose a particular setting in which to work, but then have the opportunity to select a supervisor. Some trainees even seek out supervision from a particular person with whom they want to work.

Given the choice of supervisor, how should you determine who would provide the best supervision to you? There are a number of important factors to consider. The primary factor should be the kind of experience you want to gain. Do you want to work with children, adolescents, adults, or the elderly? Do you want to gain experience in a particular area, like eating disorders or marital therapy? Do you want to work in a hospital, a community mental health clinic, a college counseling center, a private practice, or maybe even a prison? Each time you have the opportunity to select a new clinical training experience, give thought to what sort of experience you would like to gain. Then select a supervisor who can help you to gain these experiences.

An important factor to consider, of course, is the orientation of the supervisor. While this book has been geared toward CBT, most individuals over the course of their training will (and should) seek out broader experiences. Perhaps you would like to obtain training in psychodynamic therapy, interpersonal therapy, or emotion-focused therapy. It is important to seek out a supervisor who ascribes to the orientation to which you would like to be exposed and who is familiar with the scientific basis of the treatment techniques.

Another factor to consider is how skilled the individual is at supervising trainees. It is difficult to define what makes for a skilled supervisor. In general, however, it is important to find someone who is a good teacher, who has time for his or her supervisees, and who is respectful of boundaries. Furthermore, supervision is best handled when supervisors have a sense of how to balance giving adequate guidance and providing trainees with the opportunity to take an active role in making treatment decisions. Good supervisors will know how to adjust this balance as trainees become more skilled at assessing and treating clients.

The best way to learn if a supervisor has these attributes is to ask around. If you know trainees who have worked with the individual previously, ask about their experiences. If you do not know anyone who has worked with the supervisor previously, ask the supervisor for the names of some former trainees whom you can contact to ask about their experiences. Most supervisors will be open to this request—for those who are not, you may want to consider what is underlying this hesitancy.

Of course, another excellent way to get a sense of potential supervisors is to meet with them. Ask the individual about his or her work (e.g., orientation, kinds of clients that he or she sees) and what kinds of opportunities you will have working with him or her. Ask how much supervision you will receive and how supervision will be structured (e.g., individual supervision, group supervision, or a combination of the two). The way that this information is delivered to you will give you a sense of the way that the supervisor treats his or her trainees. Again, it is hard to articulate what you should be looking for—but in general, it is ideal to find supervisors who are enthusiastic about their work and eager to impart their knowledge to trainees, but also open to learning from trainees in return. A strong alliance between supervisor and trainee can be an important tool in achieving the various goals of supervision, including increasing the trainee's clinical competence.

Defining What the Relationship Will Entail

Once you and a supervisor agree to establish a supervisory relationship, it is important to articulate what this relationship will entail. The first thing to decide is how often supervision will be held and what will occur during the meetings. It is also important to discuss what kind of initial training you will receive (e.g., training in particular assessments or types of therapeutic interventions) and to agree on your caseload. You will have other responsibilities, and it is important that you not be swamped with cases to the detriment of your other duties. It is also important that you and your supervisor discuss how your work will be evaluated, on an ongoing basis as well as at the end of the training experience.

METHODS OF SUPERVISION

The way that supervision is carried out varies greatly from setting to setting and from supervisor to supervisor. In the following section, we discuss these various methods of supervision and suggest ways in which trainees can get the most out of their supervisory experiences.

Individual versus Group Supervision

Some supervisors meet individually with trainees; others meet with a number of trainees at a time in a group setting. Typically, individual meetings occur once per week and last for at least 1 hour. Group meetings should last at least 2 hours and often last longer, depending on the number of trainees being supervised and how many cases each trainee has. Supervisors who hold group supervision are usually open to trainees also arranging one-on-one meetings as needed.

Individual and group supervision each have advantages and disadvantages. Ideally, all trainees would participate in both, thus garnering the benefits of both. In individual supervision, trainees receive more attention than they would in a group setting. Individual supervision also affords greater opportunity for mentorship from the supervisor in terms of career choices, decisions about subsequent clinical experiences and supervisors, and so forth. In individual supervision, it is likely that more time will be dedicated to each case and that trainees will receive supervision on a greater number of cases since they do not need to share their supervision time with others.

In group supervision, trainees are typically asked to select difficult cases to present and are usually allotted less time to discuss each case. Despite these limitations, group supervision affords the opportunity to hear about many more cases than the ones that you are directly treating. This provides more exposure to different clinical presentations, tricky diagnostic issues, case conceptualization, treatment planning, and issues related to the treatment process.

Some trainees find it very stressful to be evaluated and given feedback in a group setting. There are various ways to deal with these concerns. First, trainees can reframe their perceptions. A wonderful thing about group supervision is that it affords the opportunity to get feedback from not only the supervisor, but also from peers at various levels of training. At times, supervision might feel like being in front of a firing squad, but if the anxiety about being evaluated can be put aside, it is likely that getting feedback from more than one person will be extremely beneficial in your development as a clinician.

Certainly, it can sometimes be appropriate to have a talk with people who deliver feedback in an overly direct or critical manner. It can be helpful to let them know why their behavior is difficult for you ("When I start to show videos of my cases, I feel like you begin to criticize my work before you've seen a long enough segment to see how things unfold") and how they can change their behavior to be more beneficial ("It would be helpful if we could watch slightly longer segments of tapes before we start to discuss the case. I feel like your feedback would be much more beneficial to me that way").

In sum, individual and group supervision both have advantages and disadvantages. It is up to trainees to try to get experiences that they feel are missing in the supervision arrangement that they have. For example, if you have a particularly difficult case that is sometimes not covered in group supervision, you should try to set up an individual meeting each week until it feels like the case is on the right track. Similarly, if you are in individual supervision, but feel that you would benefit from hearing about a greater number of cases, an informal peer supervision meeting can be arranged with other trainees.

Sharing Your Work with Your Supervisor

Supervision is only as useful as trainees make it. The responsibility is on trainees to come to supervision prepared to share their work with their supervisor in order to get the kind of feedback and advice that they need. In the next section, we discuss various methods of sharing your work, outlining the pros and cons of each, and explaining how to best prepare for supervision meetings so that you can get the most out of them.

Self-Report Method

The self-report method is the most commonly used method of supervision. This method generally involves the trainee giving an account of what happened during an assessment with a new client or during the most recent session of therapy with an ongoing client. Although the self-report method sounds like it involves little preparation on the part of the trainee, this is certainly not the case.

Before each meeting, compile a list of all of your clients, note whether or not you had a session since the last supervision meeting, and make a brief note about what you did in the session. Consider how your case conceptualization has developed and changed from session to session, and how this "updated" understanding has impacted your treatment plan. In some settings, it is also important to come ready to give a quantitative assessment of how the client is doing—for example, in a depression treatment clinic, you might be asked to report the client's Beck Depression Inventory score for that week. Perhaps most importantly, you should also come to supervision with questions that you would like to ask your supervisor or concerns that you would like to bring up. In addition to bringing this summary sheet with you to meetings, you should also bring the entire chart. This serves two purposes. First, your supervisor might request some additional information that you do not know offhand but could easily locate in the chart. Second, at the end of the supervision meeting, supervisors must sign trainees' progress notes, and the best way to ensure that this is done is to bring the chart along.

Taping

Many supervisors use video and audiotaping in their supervisory practices. Both of these allow for greater access to the therapy sessions and eliminate the bias inherent in the self-report method. Despite the clear benefits of taping, many trainees dislike this method. Being taped can increase self-focus during the session, making it more difficult to concentrate on the client. Furthermore, viewing tapes in the presence of others can be anxiety-provoking. Fortunately, this discomfort usually dissipates quickly once you become accustomed to taping sessions and to seeing or hearing yourself on tape.

To get the most benefit out of this method, trainees should listen to or view tapes on their own before supervision meetings. Supervision will be most effective if you write down specific questions and concerns and if you note the tape location of relevant segments. These "cued" parts of the tape can then be given to your supervisor to view before supervision meetings or can be shown during meetings. Generally, supervisors will not have time to listen to every tape for all their trainees each week, so the responsibility is on the individual clinician to cue the supervisor to parts of the session with which they require help. From time to time trainees have very difficult sessions and find it virtually impossible to find a specific segment of the session to show to the supervisor. In these cases, supervisors are sometimes willing to watch the whole tape and then discuss it with the trainee.

A common question that comes up regarding supervision is whether only "difficult" segments of tapes should be brought in to meetings or whether "good" segments should be brought in as well. Although we certainly do not want to focus only on the negative, supervision time is limited and should generally be used to seek guidance on difficult clinical issues. In group supervision, however, it can be helpful for trainees to occasionally bring in "good" parts of sessions. Perhaps you explained a concept very well, or dealt very effectively with a difficult clinical issue, or did a behavioral experiment with a client that resulted in some very positive changes for them. Showing these segments to the group can be very educational for other trainees.

Live Observation

Supervision can also take place via live observation. Some supervisors even "cotreat" clients with a trainee. This allows the supervisor to observe the trainee "in action" and affords the opportunity to provide guidance as the session progresses. Supervisors can also watch therapy sessions from behind a one-way mirror, either providing feedback as the session takes place (via a "bug in the ear") or immediately after the session is over. As with "cotherapy," a distinct advantage of this approach is that the supervisor can see what transpires in the therapy session in real time. Yet, similar to video and audiotaping, live observation can be anxiety-provoking for beginning clinicians. As we have already mentioned, this anxiety tends to dissipate over time. Once it does, live observation can serve as a very dynamic and helpful method of supervision.

Using a Variety of Methods

Although we have discussed distinct methods of supervision here, most supervisors employ multiple methods when they supervise trainees. Supervisors are also typically quite open to suggestions about the process of supervision. For example, if you are working with a supervisor who typically does not have trainees tape their sessions, but you believe that this method would be helpful, suggest it. It is important that trainees get the most possible out of training experiences; taking an assertive stance in the supervisory relationship can have very positive benefits.

ROADBLOCKS IN THE SUPERVISORY RELATIONSHIP

In the next section, we will discuss difficult situations than can arise in the supervisory relationship and how to resolve these situations. Although each situation is resolved in slightly different ways, a general rule to follow is to keep the lines of communication open between supervisors and trainees. Very often, particularly in settings where there are numerous trainees, concerns about the supervisory relationship are "dealt with" by griping to fellow trainees about the many faults of the supervisor. There is no doubt that seeking support from peers is helpful. It can make you feel less alone and more supported and can be helpful for generating solutions to difficult problems. Nevertheless, there can be no replacement for directly speaking to a supervisor and trying to work on the problems in a collaborative way.

Difficulties with the Way Cases Are Understood and Treated

"My Supervisor Thinks He's the Clinician"

The greatest skill of supervision is to balance giving guidance to trainees with letting them "fly" on their own, so to speak, taking responsibility for their clients' care. Some supervisors, even when trainees become more advanced, have a difficult time finding this balance, providing too much guidance and not enough independence. This is a troubling situation for beginning clinicians. This ongoing heavy-handedness can make beginning clinicians feel that they lack skills. Furthermore, if trainees do not heed the advice of the supervisor and go with their own sense of how a session should proceed, they might face reprimand.

SOLVING THE PROBLEM

This situation should be handled differently depending on in the amount of training you have received. If you are just beginning to do therapy (or just beginning to do a new kind of therapy), it is best to follow the advice offered. Later in your training, however, this issue should be brought up with the supervisor, particularly if he or she reprimands you for not following his or her guidance to a tee. Rather than criticizing the supervisor for his or her behavior, let the supervisor know how this behavior affects you. Tell the supervisor that in taking control of the therapy, he or she makes you feel as if your ability to treat clients and make clinical decisions is not being developed. Be open to criticism—ask if there is anything you are doing or not doing that makes your supervisor believe that you are not ready or able to treat clients with less direct input. If there is no specific concern, let the supervisor know that you would like to have the opportunity to work increasingly independently, while still benefiting from his or her mentorship.

"My Supervisor and I Have Conflicting Orientations"

In the course of our training, we sometimes have to work with supervisors who do not share our theoretical orientation to understanding and treating psychological difficulties. This sometimes occurs when trainees are assigned a supervision experience, rather than being able to select one based on their interests. Trainees might feel confused about whether or not they should adopt the orientation of the supervisor. If they do, they will obviously have to go against their own beliefs on how to best understand and treat psychological difficulties. If they do not, they risk reprimand from the supervisor. Furthermore, if trainees adhere to their own orientation when being supervised by someone of another orientation, they risk getting inadequate supervision.

SOLVING THE PROBLEM

The best way to deal with this confusion is to discuss it with the supervisor. It is likely that most will want trainees to treat clients in a way that is congruent with the supervisor's theoretical orientation. This is not necessarily a negative outcome. In fact, learning to do different kinds of therapy can ultimately make you a better clinician. Skills picked up from different supervisory experiences definitely influence your work, regardless of the orientation to which you eventually ascribe. Furthermore, gaining diverse supervisory experiences can alter your career path in very positive ways. For example, one of our colleagues was exposed almost exclusively to CBT throughout her training until a practicum during her final year of graduate school that was much more psychodynamic in orientation. This individual found the experience of doing psychodynamic therapy extremely enjoyable and much more in line with how she understood psychological difficulties. She ended up pursuing further training in psychodynamic therapy and continued on this path as her career got underway.

At times, trainees seek out a particular supervisor because of his or her orientation and then come to realize that the supervisor does not ascribe to the orientation to the degree that they had expected. For example, a trainee might seek out a CBT supervisor and find that he or she often provides feedback and advice that is more psychodynamic in nature. In such situations, trainees feel that they are not getting the kind of training that they had wanted. Some supervisors will be very receptive to this kind of feedback. While they might practice in a more eclectic style, they might be able to stay more focused in the supervisory relationship (e.g., following the cognitive-behavioral approach to understanding and treating clients' difficulties). Other supervisors will be less receptive, wanting the trainee to follow their advice even if it does not map onto the trainee's understanding of what a CBT clinician should do. This is a difficult situation, since in many cases trainees cannot discontinue a supervisory relationship midsemester and switch to someone more well suited to their needs. In most cases, it is best to stick with a training experience for the agreed-upon time and see what can be learned from it. Even a very negative experience can have a positive outcome, whether it be learning how you do *not* want to do therapy or learning how to better select supervisors for the next supervisory relationship.

Difficulties with Supervisor–Trainee Rapport

"I'm Scared of Being Judged Negatively by My Supervisor"

Perhaps the biggest concern for trainees in the context of the supervisory relationship is the prospect of evaluation by supervisors. This concern is not unfounded, since supervision typically involves receiving "constructive criticism." Often supervisors are so focused on providing it that they forget to offer even the slightest bit of praise. This absence of positives is exacerbated by the fact that, in supervision, we tend to bring in segments of therapy sessions that were problematic. Trainees often leave supervision meetings feeling as if their work was terribly bad and that they have no hope of ever being a good clinician. Furthermore, a particularly trying supervision meeting can make trainees very anxious about the next one. This can negatively affect the therapy, since trainees will be so focused on doing the "right thing" for fear of being reprimanded during supervision that they will not be able to attend to the client.

SOLVING THE PROBLEM

One way to deal with fear of negative evaluation is to reframe the way in which you perceive the supervisory experience. Supervision, both from supervisors and from peers, can be amazingly educational, even if at times it is hard to swallow. Beginning clinicians need to develop a thick skin and remember that feedback is not intended as a personal affront, but rather as a means to help them grow. When beginning clinicians learn to be in supervision meetings and not take feedback personally, they get a great deal more out of it.

In our experience, another reason that beginning clinicians may dread being evaluated by their supervisors is because the grounds for evaluation are elusive and unclear. What happens when you explain a concept incorrectly? How about treating a client who does not improve? What happens when a client drops out of therapy? Do these events lead to poor grades or some other negative outcome? The best way to deal with these worries is to establish with supervisors, right from the start of a supervisory experience, what the grounds for evaluation are. Evaluation of therapy skills is difficult. It is best to not get too distressed about giving one poor explanation, having an occasional client who is nonresponsive to treatment, or having a few patients drop out of treatment prematurely. Supervisors typically look at the "bigger picture"—whether trainees put effort into their work, behave in an ethical and compassionate manner, and show improvement in therapy skills over the course of a training experience.

"My Supervisor Has No Time for Me"

In contrast to overinvolved supervisors, some supervisors simply do not have time for their trainees. They may miss supervision meetings or refuse to set them up at all. They may be unavailable to trainees outside of set supervision times, even for very difficult clinical situations. When such supervisors do meet with trainees, meetings tend to be very rushed and often interrupted by phone calls or by other people dropping by the office. Regardless of the exact nature of the problem, trainees are left with inadequate supervision.

This is problematic for a number of different reasons. First and foremost, it results in poorer-quality care for clients. As we have already noted, no supervisor expects trainees to begin a training experience already possessing all of the skills that they need to do good clinical work. It is difficult to imagine a training experience (even a relatively poor one) where trainees do not learn something to benefit their clients. However, supervision meetings must be held for these benefits to be realized.

Along with poor-quality care for clients, poor supervision also results in a poor learning experience for trainees. Trainees will come away from such experiences feeling as if they have not acquired new skills or knowledge. They will also miss out on the opportunity for mentorship. Furthermore, they will not have the opportunity to learn the skill of supervision—which is best learned through our own supervision experiences when we are trainees.

SOLVING THE PROBLEM

One of the most difficult things about solving the problem of the unavailable supervisor is getting him or her to commit to meeting to have this discussion. This is a good time to practice your assertiveness skills—insist that you must meet and that the meeting must occur as soon as possible. Be open about your concerns—let the supervisor know that you feel as if you are "paddling your own canoe" and that you feel that more frequent and reliable supervision is essential. While the responsibility is certainly on the supervisor to figure out how to find time for trainees, you can come in with some suggestions. Perhaps better supervision could be given if meetings were held at a different time, or if cases were occasionally discussed by phone, or if plans were in place for a backup supervisor to take over when your main supervisor is too busy, for example. Some supervisors will be responsive to your requests for better supervision and will become more diligent when they realize the impact that their behavior has on clients and on you.

When this message does not result in a change in behavior, however, trainees can remind supervisors of the possible consequences of their negligence. Ultimately, supervisors are ethically and legally responsible for your clients' welfare. If they are not involved in clients' care, and something happens to a client, their license and their professional livelihood is on the line. If this does not effectively change their behavior, it is in your best interest, and your clients', to discontinue the supervisory relationship and make new arrangements.

"My Supervisor and I Disagree on Moral/Ethical Issues"

Clients often present material during therapy sessions that may be cause for alarm. For example, clients will occasionally report feeling suicidal, have sexual thoughts about their clinician, bring in gifts for their clinician, report participating in illegal activities, and have knowledge of the mistreatment of a child. In each of these situations, consultation with a supervisor is obviously necessary. It is possible for a trainee and supervisor to have different opinions about how to resolve such issues. For example, a trainee might believe that a client's suicidal ideation is not genuine, while the supervisor might believe that it is.

SOLVING THE PROBLEM

In such situations, it is obviously important for the trainee and supervisor to discuss their differences. Additionally, it is important for students to remember that the ultimate ethical, moral, legal, and professional responsibility for the client remains with the supervisor. Therefore, in almost all cases the supervisor's decisions should be followed and respected. In the event that a discrepancy of clinical judgment cannot be resolved, the trainee should ask the supervisor if they might consult with another individual, most typically the clinic director or the director of clinical training. Experienced clinicians often resolve ethical or moral dilemmas by consulting with colleagues, and most supervisors will be receptive to this arrangement. If your supervisor is not receptive, it might still be worth speaking to the clinic director or the director of clinical training—not about the case per se, but rather about the supervisor's reluctance to consult with colleagues about difficult clinical issues.

"My Supervisor Is Trying to Be My Therapist"

Clinicians should not use the supervisory relationship as a means of getting therapy for themselves. Similarly, it is not appropriate for the supervisor to take on the role of therapist. This is a sometimes difficult line to draw, as it is certainly reasonable for the supervisor to comment or inquire about the trainee's behavior, both as a beginning therapist and as a trainee. However, this establishes a dual relationship in which the supervisor serves as both supervisor and clinician. Knowing a great deal about their trainees' personal lives can bias the supervisor's evaluation of their work, and there are limits that must be observed (see APA code 7.05b).

SOLVING THE PROBLEM

The responsibility is most often on the trainee to keep personal issues out of the supervisory relationship. However, it is sometimes the supervisor who initiates the therapeutic stance in the supervisory relationship. While trainees can try to direct attention away from their own issues in supervision meetings, this sort of difficulty is often best resolved by speaking about it directly with the supervisor. If this approach fails, supervisees might request a meeting with the supervisor and the supervisor's supervisor or another colleague to resolve the issue. Only if no reasonable solution is found should other alternatives, such as terminating a practicum experience, be considered.

"My Supervisor Is Behaving Inappropriately toward Me"

One of the most difficult situations for beginning clinicians to handle is when supervisors behave in an inappropriate manner. A number of researchers have reported on the high incidence of sexual harassment on the part of supervisors (Fitzgerald et al., 1988). Supervisors might be very complimentary of their trainees' appearance or manner of dress, might ask trainees personal questions (e.g., about their relationship status or about issues in the trainees' relationships), and might even do more overtly inappropriate things, like make sexual advances. All of these behaviors make trainees extremely uncomfortable and leave them feeling unsure of how best to resolve the situation.

There are a number of reasons why this type of situation is so difficult to resolve. First and foremost, there is a power differential in the supervisory relationship. The supervisor has control over your grades and, in a sense, over your future. We depend on supervisors as people who will serve as references when we apply for further training and for jobs and who will sign off on documents necessary during the process of getting licensed. Beginning clinicians worry that if they do not conform to a supervisor's demands, they will not reap the benefits of their hard work.

Many beginning clinicians who face this difficult situation also feel unsure of where to turn for guidance. In many clinic settings and academic departments, staff members and faculty seem to be friendly with one another, and trainees might wonder if there is anyone that they can turn to for help who will respect their desire for confidentiality. Another concern is whether trainees' reports will be taken seriously. A major problem with this type of inappropriate behavior is that there is often no "proof" that it happened. Many trainees worry that if they report the inappropriate behavior, they will not be believed.

SOLVING THE PROBLEM

In light of these concerns, making the decision of how to deal with this type of situation is often quite trying. Throughout this book, we have recommended that the best way to deal with difficult situations in the therapeutic relationship and in the supervisory relationship is to be direct—tell the individual in question what the problem is, why it is difficult for you, and how the situation might best be solved. It is difficult to puzzle out whether this would be an effective way to deal with inappropriate behavior on the part of a supervisor. While trainees want the inappropriate behavior to stop, they do not want to run the risk of making their situations even worse.

In some situations, trainees might sense that the supervisor will be open to feedback and that it is worth telling the supervisor how they would like him or her to change. In many situations, however, this will not be the case, and it will be necessary to take the issue to a superior such as the clinic director, the director of clinical training, or the department chairman. What trainees must do is consider whether to deal with the situation during their training experience, once it is over, or never at all.

We encourage trainees to deal with situations in which supervisors behave inappropriately. It is very likely that the supervisor has behaved this way in the past toward other trainees and will continue to behave this way toward future trainees. This knowledge has some important implications. First, it might be that when you report inappropriate behavior, your report will not be the first received. In fact, your report might corroborate others and make clearer the case against an unethical supervisor. Second, your report could protect future trainees who might find themselves in a similar situation.

We are then left with the decision of whether to act immediately or once a training experience is complete. In many cases, it can be best to wait until the training experience is complete. If the supervisor's inappropriate behaviors are very subtle (e.g., commenting on your appearance, asking you personal questions, etc.), this might be the best way to proceed. Immediate action is the better alternative under a few conditions. The most obvious is when your evaluation is going to depend on whether or not you comply with the supervisor's requests. If the supervisor says that he will fail you and write you terrible reference letters if you do not sleep with him, immediate action must be taken. Similarly, if you feel unsafe in any way or worry that your level of discomfort within supervision meetings is having a negative impact on your ability to treat clients, it is best that immediate action be taken.

One general rule of thumb to follow in such cases is to document everything. While it would be unethical to surreptitiously tape record supervision meetings, it can be very helpful to make a record of what went on in each supervision meeting once it is over. This record can then be used when a complaint is made. Particularly if you wait until the end of a training experience to do so, some people (particularly the accused supervisor) might doubt the accuracy of your complaints. Your case will be much stronger if incidents are documented as they occur.

FOCUSING ON THE POSITIVE

As in other chapters of this book, this chapter has focused on the challenges that come up in the lives of clinicians. A by-product of this focus might be a negativistic tone. Keep in mind, however, that the majority of supervisory experiences are positive. Many of us feel indebted to a particular supervisor who not only taught us a great deal about being a clinician, but also served as a mentor as we set out on our career paths. When supervisory relationships are wrapping up, most supervisors evaluate their trainees. It can also be very helpful (and required in some settings) for trainees to evaluate their supervisors. Most supervisors appreciate some constructive criticism and, certainly, all supervisors like to hear how they were helpful and what trainees got out of the training experience.

Appendix A

■ ■ ■

RECOMMENDED READINGS IN COGNITIVE-BEHAVIORAL THERAPY

THEORY AND RESEARCH

Alford, B. A., & Beck, A. T. (1997). *The integrative power of cognitive therapy.* New York: Guilford Press.

Asmundson, G. J. G., Taylor, S., & Cox, B. J. (Eds.). (2001). *Health anxiety: Clinical and research perspectives on hypochondriasis and related disorders.* Chichester, UK: Wiley.

Beck, A. T. (1999). *Cognitive aspects of personality disorders and their relation to syndromal disorders: A psychoevolutionary aspect.* In C. R. Cloninger (Ed.), *Personality and psychopathology* (pp. 411–429). Washington, DC: American Psychiatric Press.

Beck, A. T. (1999). *Prisoners of hate: The cognitive basis of anger, hostility, and violence.* New York: HarperCollins.

Butler, A. C., & Beck, J. S. (2000). Cognitive therapy outcomes: A review of meta-analyses. *Journal of the Norwegian Psychological Association, 37,* 1–9.

Clark, D. A., Beck, A. T., & Alford, B. A. (1999). *Scientific foundations of cognitive therapy and therapy of depression.* New York: Wiley.

Gelder, M. (1997). The scientific foundations of cognitive behavior therapy. In D. M. Clark & C. G. Fairburn (Eds.), *Science and practice of cognitive behaviour therapy* (pp. 27–46). New York: Oxford University Press.

Hollon, S. D., & Beck, A. T. (1994). Cognitive and cognitive-behavioral therapies. In A. E. Bergin & S. L. Garfield (Eds.), *Handbook of psychotherapy and behavior change* (4th ed., pp. 428–466). New York: Wiley.

Ingram, R. E., Miranda, J., & Segal, Z. V. (1999). *Cognitive vulnerability to depression.* New York: Guilford Press.

Leahy, R. L. (2003). *Psychology and the economic mind: Cognitive processes and conceptualization.* New York: Springer.

Adapted by permission of Judith S. Beck from a list compiled by the Beck Institute for Cognitive Therapy and Research (*www.beckinstitute.org*).

Leahy, R. L. (Ed.). (2004). *Contemporary cognitive therapy: Theory, research, and practice*. New York: Guilford Press.

Neenan, M., Dryden, W., & Dryden, C. (2000). *Essential cognitive therapy*. London: Whurr.

Rosner, J. (2002). *Cognitive therapy and dreams*. New York: Springer.

Taylor, S. (Ed.). (1999). *Anxiety sensitivity: Theory, research, and treatment of the fear of anxiety*. Mahwah, NJ: Erlbaum.

Taylor, S. (Ed.). (2004). *Advances in the treatment of posttraumatic stress disorder: Cognitive-behavioral perspectives*. New York: Springer.

Wright, J. (Ed.). (2004). *Review of psychiatry: Vol. 23. Cognitive-behavior therapy*. Washington, DC: American Psychiatric Press.

CLINICAL APPLICATIONS: GENERAL

Beck, J. S. (1995). *Cognitive therapy: Basics and beyond*. New York: Guilford Press.

Dobson, K. S. (Ed.). (1999). *Handbook of cognitive-behavioral therapies* (2nd ed.). New York: Guilford Press.

Freeman, A., Pretzer, J., Fleming, B., & Simon, K. M. (2004). *Clinical applications of cognitive therapy* (2nd ed.). New York: Springer.

Leahy, R. L. (2003). *Cognitive therapy techniques: A practitioner's guide*. New York: Guilford Press.

Ludgate, J. W. (1995). *Maximizing psychotherapeutic gains and preventing relapse*. Sarasota, FL: Professional Resource Press.

McMullin, R. E. (1999). *The new handbook of cognitive therapy techniques*. New York: Norton.

Needleman, L. D. (1999). *Cognitive case conceptualization: A guidebook for practitioners*. Mahwah, NJ: Erlbaum.

Nezu, A., Nezu, C. M., & Lombardo, E. (2004). *Cognitive-behavioral case formulation and treatment design: A problem-solving approach*. New York: Springer.

O'Donohue, W., Fisher, J., & Hayes, S. (2004). *Cognitive behavior therapy: Applying empirically supported techniques in your practice*. New York: Wiley.

Padesky, C. A., & Greenberger, D. (1995). *Clinician's guide to mind over mood*. New York: Guilford Press.

Persons, J. B. (1989). *Cognitive therapy in practice: A case formulation approach*. New York: Norton.

Schuyler, D. (2003). *Cognitive therapy: A practical guide*. New York: Norton.

Wells, A. (2002). *Emotional disorders and metacognition: Innovative cognitive therapy*. New York: Wiley.

CLINICAL APPLICATIONS: BOOKS ON SPECIFIC DISORDERS, PROBLEMS, OR POPULATIONS

Anxiety Disorders

Antony, M. M., & Swinson, R. P. (2000). *Phobic disorders and panic in adults: A guide to assessment and treatment*. Washington, DC: American Psychological Association.

Beck, A. T., Emery, G., & Greenberg, R. (1985). *Anxiety disorders and phobias: A cognitive perspective.* New York: Basic Books.

Clark, D. A. (2004). *Cognitive-behavioral therapy for OCD.* New York: Guilford Press.

Foa, E. B., & Rothbaum, B. O. (2001). *Treating the trauma of rape: Cognitive-behavioral therapy for PTSD.* New York: Guilford Press.

Follette, V. M., Ruzek, J. I., & Abueg, F. R. (1998). *Cognitive-behavioral therapies for trauma.* New York: Guilford Press.

Frost, R. O., & Steketee, G. (Eds.). (2002). *Cognitive approaches to obsessions and compulsions: Theory, assessment, and treatment.* Oxford, UK: Elsevier.

Heimberg, R. G., & Becker, R. E. (2002). *Cognitive-behavioral group therapy for social phobia: Basic mechanisms and clinical applications.* New York: Guilford Press.

Heimberg, R. G., Turk, C. L., & Mennin, D. S. (Eds.). (2004). *Generalized anxiety disorder: Advances in research and practice.* New York: Guilford Press.

Najavits, L. M. (2001). *Seeking safety: A treatment manual for PTSD and substance abuse.* New York: Guilford Press.

Rygh, J. R., & Sanderson, W. C. (2004). *Treating generalized anxiety disorder: Evidence-based strategies, tools, and techniques.* New York: Guilford Press.

Taylor, S. (2000). *Understanding and treating panic disorder: Cognitive-behavioural approaches.* New York: Wiley.

Taylor, S. (Ed.). (2004). *Advances in the treatment of posttraumatic stress disorder: Cognitive-behavioral perspectives.* New York: Springer.

Taylor, S., & Asmundson, G. J. G. (2004). *Treating health anxiety: A cognitive-behavioral approach.* New York: Guilford Press.

Bipolar Disorder

Basco, M. R., & Rush, A. J. (2005). *Cognitive-behavioral therapy for bipolar disorder* (2nd ed.). New York: Guilford Press.

Johnson, S. L., & Leahy, R. L. (Eds.). (2003). *Psychological treatment of bipolar disorder.* New York: Guilford Press.

Lam, D. H., Jones, S. H., Hayward, P., & Bright, J. A. (1999). *Cognitive therapy for bipolar disorder: A therapist's guide to concepts, methods and practice.* New York: Wiley.

Newman, C. F., Leahy, R. L., Beck, A. T., Reilly-Harrington, N. A., & Gyulai, L. (2002). *Bipolar disorder: A cognitive therapy approach.* Washington, DC: American Psychological Association.

Children

Albano, A. M., & Kearney, C. A. (2000). *When children refuse school: A cognitive behavioral therapy approach: Therapist guide.* San Antonio, TX: Psychological Corporation.

Braswell, L., & Bloomquist, M. L. (1991). *Cognitive-behavioral therapy with ADHD children: Child, family, and school interventions.* New York: Guilford Press.

Deblinger, E., & Heflin, A. H. (1996). *Treating sexually abused children and their nonoffending parents: A cognitive behavioral approach.* Thousand Oaks, CA: Sage.

Friedberg, R. D., Crosby, L. E., Friedberg, B. A., & Friedberg, R. J. (2001). *Therapeutic exercises for children: Guided self-discovery using cognitive-behavioral techniques.* Sarasota, FL: Professional Resource Press.

Friedberg, R., & McClure, J. (2001). *Clinical practice of cognitive therapy with children and adolescents: The nuts and bolts.* New York: Guilford Press.

Kendall, P. C. (Ed.). (2000). *Child and adolescent therapy: Cognitive-behavioral procedures* (2nd ed.). New York: Guilford Press.

March, J. S., & Mulle, K. (1998). *OCD in children and adolescents: A cognitive-behavioral treatment manual.* New York: Guilford Press.

Reinecke, M. A., Dattilio, F. M., & Freeman, A. (Eds.). (2003). *Cognitive therapy with children and adolescents: A casebook for clinical practice* (2nd ed.). New York: Guilford Press.

Stallard, P. (2002). *Think good—feel good: A cognitive behaviour therapy workbook for children.* Druin, Victoria, Australia: Halsted Press.

Temple, S. D. (1997). *Brief therapy of adolescent depression.* Sarasota, FL: Professional Resources Press.

Depression and Suicide

Beck, A. T., Rush, A. J., Shaw, B. F., & Emery, G. (1979). *Cognitive therapy of depression.* New York: Guilford Press.

Freeman, A., & Reinecke, M. (1994). *Cognitive therapy of suicidal behavior.* New York: Springer.

McCullough, J. P. (1999). *Treatment for chronic depression: Cognitive behavioral analysis system of psychotherapy.* New York: Guilford Press.

Moore, R., & Garland, A. (2003). *Cognitive therapy for chronic and persistent depression.* New York: Wiley.

Papageorgiou, C., & Wells, A. (2003). *Depressive rumination: Nature, theory and treatment.* New York: Wiley.

Persons, J. B., Davidson, J., & Tomkins, M. A. (2001). *Essential components of cognitive-behavioral therapy for depression.* Washington, DC: American Psychological Association.

Rudd, M. D., Joiner, T., & Rajab, M. H. (2001). *Treating suicidal behavior: An effective, time-limited approach.* New York: Guilford Press.

Segal, Z. V., Williams, J., Mark, G., & Teasdale, J. D. (2002). *Mindfulness-based cognitive therapy for depression: A new approach to preventing relapse.* New York: Guilford Press.

Eating Disorders

Cooper, Z., Fairburn, C. G., & Hawker, D. M. (2003). *Cognitive-behavioral treatment of obesity: A clinician's guide.* New York: Guilford Press.

Garner, D. M., Vitousek, K. M., & Pike, K. M. (1997). Cognitive-behavioral therapy for anorexia nervosa. In D. M. Garner & P. E. Garfinkel (Eds.), *Handbook of treatment for eating disorders* (2nd ed., pp. 94–144). New York: Guilford Press.

Group Therapy

Free, M. E. (2000). *Cognitive therapy in groups: Guidelines and resources for practice.* New York: Wiley.

White, J., & Freeman, A. (2000). *Cognitive-behavioral group therapy for specific problems and populations.* Washington, DC: American Psychological Association.

Marriage and Family Problems

Baucom, D. H., & Bozicas, G. D. (1990). *Cognitive behavioral marital therapy.* New York: Brunner/Mazel.

Dattilio, F. M. (1998). *Case studies in couple and family therapy: Systemic and cognitive perspectives.* New York: Guilford Press.

Dattilio, F. M., & Padesky, C. A. (1990). *Cognitive therapy with couples.* Sarasota, FL: Professional Resources Press.

Epstein, N. B., & Baucom, D. H. (2002). *Enhanced cognitive-behavioral therapy for couples: A contextual approach.* Washington, DC: American Psychological Association.

Epstein, N. E., Schlesinger, S. E., & Dryden, W. (Eds.). (1988). *Cognitive-behavioral therapy with families.* New York: Brunner/Mazel.

Medical Problems

Crawford, I., & Fishman, B. (Eds.). (1996). *Psychosocial interventions for HIV disease: A stage-focused and culture specific approach (cognitive behavioral therapy).* Northvale, NJ: Jason Aronson.

Henry, J. L., & Wilson, P. H. (2000). *Psychological management of chronic tinnitus: A cognitive-behavioral approach.* New York: Pearson Allyn & Bacon.

Moorey, S., & Greer, S. (2002). *Cognitive behaviour therapy for people with cancer.* New York: Oxford University Press.

Segal, Z. V., Toner, B. B., Shelagh, D. E., & Myran, D. (1999). *Cognitive-behavioral treatment of irritable bowel syndrome: The brain–gut connection.* New York: Guilford Press.

Thorn, B. E. (2004). *Cognitive therapy for chronic pain: A step-by-step guide.* New York: Guilford Press.

White, C. A. (2001). *Cognitive behaviour therapy for chronic medical problems.* Chichester, UK: Wiley.

Winterowd, C., Beck, A., & Gruener, D. (2003). *Cognitive therapy with chronic pain patients.* New York: Springer.

Obsessive–Compulsive Disorder

Clark, D. A. (2004). *Cognitive-behavioral therapy for OCD.* New York: Guilford Press.

Older Adults

Laidlaw, K., Thompson, L. W., Dick-Siskin, L., & Gallagher-Thompson, D. (2003). *Cognitive behaviour therapy with older people.* Chichester, UK: Wiley.

Yost, E. B., Beutler, L. E., Corbishley, M. A., & Allender, J. R. (1987). *Group cognitive therapy: A treatment approach for depressed older adults.* New York: Pergamon.

Personality Disorders

Beck, A. T., Freeman, A., Davis, D. D., & Associates. (2003). *Cognitive therapy of personality disorders* (2nd ed.). New York: Guilford Press.

Layden, M. A., Newman, C. F., Freeman, A., & Morse, S. B. (1993). *Cognitive therapy of borderline personality disorder.* Boston: Allyn & Bacon.

Linehan, M. (1993). *Cognitive-behavioral treatment of borderline personality disorder.* New York: Guilford Press.

Smucker, M. R., & Dancu, C. V. (1999). *Cognitive behavioral treatment of adult survivors of childhood trauma: Imagery rescripting and reprocessing.* Northvale, NJ: Jason Aronson.

Sperry, L. (1999). *Cognitive behavior therapy of DSM-IV personality disorders.* New York: Brunner-Routledge.

Young, J., Klosko, J., & Weishaar, M. E. (2003). *Schema therapy: A practitioner's guide.* New York: Guilford Press.

Resistance

Leahy, R. L. (2001). *Overcoming resistance in cognitive therapy.* New York: Guilford Press.

Leahy, R. L. (2003). *Roadblocks in cognitive-behavioral therapy: Transforming challenges into opportunities for change.* New York: Guilford Press.

Substance Abuse

Beck, A. T., Wright, F. D., Newman, C. F., & Liese, B. S. (1993). *Cognitive therapy of substance abuse.* New York: Guilford Press.

Najavits, L. M. (2001). *Seeking safety: A treatment manual for PTSD and substance abuse.* New York: Guilford Press.

Thase, M. (1997). *Cognitive-behavioral therapy for substance abuse disorders.* In L. J. Dickstein, M. B. Riba, & J. M. Oldham (Eds.), *Review of psychiatry* (Vol. 16, pp. 45–72). Washington, DC: American Psychiatric Press.

Schizophrenia

Chadwick, P., Birchwood, M., & Trower, P. (1996). *Cognitive therapy of delusions, voices, and paranoia.* New York: Wiley.

French, P., & Morrison, A. (2004). *Early detection and cognitive therapy for people at high risk for psychosis: A treatment approach.* New York: Wiley.

Kingdon, D., & Turkington, D. (1994). *Cognitive-behavioral therapy of schizophrenia.* Hillside, NJ: Erlbaum.

Kingdon, D., & Turkington, D. (Eds.). (2002). *A case study guide to cognitive behavioural therapy of psychosis.* Chichester, UK: Wiley.

Marco, M. C. G., Perris, C., & Brenner, B. (Eds.). (2002). *Cognitive therapy with schizophrenic patients: The evolution of a new treatment approach.* Cambridge, MA: Hogrefe & Huber.

Morrison, A. (2002). *A casebook of cognitive therapy for psychosis.* New York: Brunner-Routledge.

Morrison, A. P. (2004). *Cognitive therapy for psychosis: A formulation-based approach.* New York: Brunner-Routledge.

Miscellaneous

Bedrosian, R. C., & Bozicas, G. (1994). *Treating family of origin problems: A cognitive approach.* New York: Guilford Press.

Freeman, A., & Dattilio, F. M. (Eds.). (2000). *Cognitive-behavioral strategies in crisis intervention* (2nd ed.). New York: Guilford Press.

Kroese, B. S., Dagnan, D., & Loumides, K. (Eds.). (1997). *Cognitive behaviour therapy for people with learning disabilities.* New York: Routledge.

Martell, C. R., Safran, S. A., & Prince, S. E. (2003). *Cognitive-behavioral therapies with lesbian, gay, and bisexual clients.* New York: Guilford Press.

Radnitz, C. L. (Ed.). (2000). *Cognitive behavioral therapy for persons with disabilities.* Northvale, NJ: Jason Aronson.

Safran, J. D., & Segal, Z. V. (1996). *Interpersonal process in cognitive therapy.* Northvale, NJ: Jason Aronson.

Wills, F., & Sanders, D. (1997). *Cognitive therapy: Transforming the image.* London: Sage.

Wright, J. H., Thase, M. E., Beck, A. T., & Ludgate, J. W. (1993). *Cognitive therapy with inpatients: Developing a cognitive milieu.* New York: Guilford Press.

CLINICAL APPLICATIONS: BOOKS COVERING MULTIPLE DISORDERS, PROBLEMS, OR POPULATIONS

Barlow, D. H. (Ed.). (2001). *Clinical handbook of psychological disorders: A step-by-step treatment manual* (3rd ed.). New York: Guilford Press.

Beck, A. T. (1976). *Cognitive therapy and the emotional disorders.* New York: International Universities Press.

Blackburn, I. M., Twaddle, V., & Associates. (1996). *Cognitive therapy in action: A practitioner's casebook.* London. Souvenier Press (Educational & Academic).

Caballo, V. E. (Ed.). (1998). *International handbook of cognitive and behavioural treatments for psychological disorders.* Oxford, UK: Elsevier Science.

Clark, D. M., & Fairburn, C. G. (Eds.). (1997). *Science and practice of cognitive behavior therapy.* New York: Oxford University Press.

Freeman, A., & Dattilio, F. M. (1992). *Comprehensive casebook of cognitive therapy.* New York: Plenum.

Freeman, A., Pretzer, J., Fleming, B., & Simon, K. M. (1990). *Clinical applications of cognitive therapy*. New York: Plenum.

Freeman, A., Simon, K. M., Beutler, L., & Arkowitz, H. (Eds.). (1989). *Comprehensive handbook of cognitive therapy*. New York: Plenum.

Granvold, D. K. (Ed.). (1998). *Cognitive and behavioral treatment: Methods and applications*. Stamford, CT: Wadsworth.

Kuehlwein, K. T., & Rosen, H. (Eds.). (1993). *Cognitive therapies in action: Evolving innovative practice*. San Francisco: Jossey-Bass.

Leahy, R. (1996). *Cognitive therapy: Basic principles and applications*. Northvale, NJ: Jason Aronson.

Leahy, R. (Ed.). (1997). *Practicing cognitive therapy: A guide to interventions*. Northvale, NJ: Jason Aronson.

Leahy, R. L., & Dowd, T. E. (Ed.). (2002). *Clinical advances in cognitive psychotherapy: Theory and application*. New York: Springer.

Leahy, R. L., & Holland, S. J. (2000). *Treatment plans and interventions for depression and anxiety disorders*. New York: Guilford Press.

Lyddon, W. J., & Jones, J. V. (Ed.). (2001). *Empirically supported cognitive therapies: Current and future applications*. New York: Springer.

Reinecke, M., & Clark, D. (Eds.). (2003). *Cognitive therapy across the lifespan: Evidence and practice*. Cambridge, UK: Cambridge University Press.

Salkovskis, P. M. (Ed.). (1996). *Frontiers of cognitive therapy*. New York: Guilford Press.

Salkovskis, P. M. (Ed.). (1996). *Trends in cognitive therapy and behavioural therapies*. New York: Wiley.

Scott, J., Williams, M. G., & Beck, A. T. (Eds.). (1989). *Cognitive therapy in clinical practice*. New York: Routledge.

Simos, G. (Ed.). (2002). *Cognitive behaviour therapy: A guide for the practicing clinician*. New York: Brunner-Routledge.

Appendix B

■ ■ ■

SUGGESTED JOURNALS AND WEBSITES

CBT-RELATED JOURNALS

Acta Psychiatrica Scandinavica
Addiction
Addictive Behaviors
American Journal of Family Therapy
American Journal of Geriatric
  Psychiatry
American Journal of Psychiatry
Anxiety, Stress and Coping
Archives of General Psychiatry
Australian and New Zealand Journal
  of Psychiatry
Behavior Modification
Behavior Therapy
Behaviour Research and Therapy
Behavioural and Cognitive
  Psychotherapy
Biological Psychiatry
Bipolar Disorders
British Journal of Clinical
  Psychology
British Journal of Psychiatry
Canadian Journal of Psychiatry
Clinical Psychology and
  Psychotherapy
Clinical Psychology Review
Clinical Psychology: Science
  and Practice
Cognitive and Behavioral Practice

Cognitive Behaviour Therapy
Cognitive Therapy and Research
Comprehensive Psychiatry
Depression and Anxiety
European Eating Disorders Review
International Journal of Eating
  Disorders
Journal of Abnormal Psychology
Journal of Affective Disorders
Journal of Anxiety Disorders
Journal of Behavior Therapy
  and Experimental Psychiatry
Journal of Clinical Psychiatry
Journal of Clinical Psychology
Journal of Cognitive Psychotherapy
Journal of Consulting and Clinical
  Psychology
Journal of Family Psychology
Journal of Marital and Family
  Therapy
Journal of Marriage and the Family
Journal of Nervous and Mental
  Disease
Journal of Personality Disorders
Journal of Psychiatric Research
Journal of Psychopathology
  and Behavioral Assessment
Journal of Studies on Alcohol

Journal of Traumatic Stress
Obesity Research
Personality and Individual Differences
Professional Psychology: Research
    and Practice
Psychiatric Clinics of North America
Psychiatry Research

Psychological Assessment
Psychological Medicine
Psychology of Addictive Behaviors
Schizophrenia Bulletin
Suicide and Life-Threatening
    Behavior

CBT-RELATED WEBSITES

Academy of Cognitive Therapy   *www.academyofct.org*

Association for Advancement of Behavior Therapy   *www.aabt.org*

Association of State and Provincial Psychology   *www.asppb.org*
    Boards (ASPPB) Roster of Member Jurisdictions

Beck Institute for Cognitive Therapy and Research   *www.beckinstitute.org*

International Association for Cognitive Psychotherapy *www.iacp.asu.edu*

REFERENCES

American Psychiatric Association. (2000). *Diagnostic and statistical manual of mental disorders* (4th ed., text rev.). Washington, DC: Author.

American Psychological Association. (2002). Ethical principles of psychologists and code of conduct. *American Psychologist, 57,* 1060–1073.

Barlow, D. H. (Ed.). (2001). *Clinical handbook of psychological disorders: A step-by-step treatment manual* (3rd ed.). New York: Guilford Press.

Basoglu, M., Marks, I. M., Kilic, C., Brewin, C. R., & Swinson, R. P. (1994). Alprazolam and exposure for panic disorder with agoraphobia attribution of improvement to medication predicts subsequent relapse. *British Journal of Psychiatry, 164,* 652–659.

Beck, A. T. (1976). *Cognitive therapy and the emotional disorders.* New York: International Universities Press.

Beck, A. T., Rush, A. J., Shaw, B., & Emery, G. (1979). *Cognitive therapy of depression.* New York: Guilford Press.

Beck, J. S. (1995). *Cognitive therapy: Basics and beyond.* New York: Guilford Press.

Brent, D. A., Perper, J. A., Mortiz, G., Allman, C., Schweers, J., Roth, C., et al. (1993). Psychiatric sequelae to the loss of an adolescent peer to suicide. *Journal of the American Academy of Child and Adolescent Psychiatry, 32,* 509–517.

Brown, T. A., DiNardo, P. A., & Barlow, D. H. (1994). Anxiety Disorders Interview Schedule for DSM-IV (ADIS-IV). San Antonio, TX: Psychological Corporation.

Burns, D. D. (1980). *Feeling good: The new mood therapy.* New York: Signet.

Canadian Psychological Association. (2000). *Canadian code of ethics for psychologists* (3rd ed.). Ottawa, Ontario: Author.

Craske, M. G., & Barlow, D. H. (2001). Panic disorder and agoraphobia. In D. H. Barlow (Ed.), *Clinical handbook of psychological disorders* (3rd ed., pp. 1–59). New York: Guilford Press.

243

Crits-Christoph, P., Baranackie, K., Kurcias, J., Beck, A. T., Carroll, K., Perry, K., Luborsky, L., McLellan, A. T., Woody, G., Thompson, L., Gallagher, D., & Zitrin, C. (1991). Meta-analysis of therapist effects in psychotherapy outcome studies. *Psychotherapy Research, 1*, 81–91.

Cukrowicz, K. C., Wingate, L. R., Driscoll, K. A., & Joiner, T. E. (2004). A standard of care for the assessment of suicide risk and associated treatment: The Florida State University psychology clinic as an example. *Journal of Contemporary Psychotherapy, 34*, 87–100.

Duberstein, P. R., & Conwell, Y. (1997). Personality disorders and completed suicide: A methodological and conceptual review. *Clinical Psychology: Science and Practice, 4*, 359–376.

First, M. B., Spitzer, R. L., Gibbon, M., & Williams, J. B. W. (1997). *Structured Clinical Interview for DSM-IV Axis I Disorders (SCID-I), Clinician Version.* Washington, DC: American Psychiatric Publishing.

Furmark, T., Tillfors, M., Marteinsdottir, I., Fischer, H., Pissiota, A., Langstroem, B., & Fredrikson, M. (2002). Common changes in cerebral blood flow in patients with social phobia treated with citalopram or cognitive-behavioral therapy. *Archives of General Psychiatry, 59*, 425–433.

Garner, D. M. (1993). Eating disorders. In A. S. Bellack & M. Hersen (Eds.), *Psychopathology in adulthood* (pp. 319–336). Needham Heights, MA: Allyn & Bacon.

Goldapple, K., Segal, Z., Garson, C., Lau, M., Bieling, P., Kennedy, S., & Mayberg, H. (2004). Modulation of cortical–limbic pathways in major depression: Treatment specific effects of cognitive behavior therapy. *Archives of General Psychiatry, 61*, 34–41.

Greenberger, D., & Padesky, C. A. (1995). *Mind over mood: Change how you feel by changing the way you think.* New York: Guilford Press.

Groth-Marnat, G. (1997). *Handbook of psychological assessment* (3rd ed.). Oxford, UK: Wiley.

Heikkinen, M. E., Isometsae, E. T., Marttunen, M. J., Aro, H. M., & Lönnqvist, J. K. (1995). Social factors in suicide. *British Journal of Psychiatry, 167*, 747–753.

Hope, D. A., Heimberg, R. G., Juster, H. R., & Turk, C. L. (2000). *Managing social anxiety: A cognitive-behavioral therapy approach.* San Antonio, TX: Psychological Corporation.

Jones, M. C. (1924). A laboratory study of fear: The case of Peter. *Pedagogical Seminary, 31*, 308–315.

Joiner, T. E., Rudd, M. D., & Rajab, M. H. (1997). The Modified Scale for Suicidal Ideation: Factors of suicidality and their relation to clinical and diagnostic variables. *Journal of Abnormal Psychology, 106*, 260–265.

Joiner, T. E., Walker, R. L., Rudd, M. D., & Jobes, D. A. (1999). Scientizing and routinizing the assessment of suicidality in outpatient practice. *Professional Psychology: Research and Practice, 30*, 447–453.

Kaplan, H. I., Sadock, B. J., & Grebb, J. A. (1994). *Kaplan and Sadock's synopsis of psychiatry: Behavioral sciences, clinical psychiatry* (7th ed.). Baltimore, MD: Williams & Wilkins.

Keijsers, G. P. J., Schaap, C. P. D. R., & Hoogduin, C. A. L. (2000). The impact of interpersonal patient and therapist behavior on outcome in cognitive-behavioral therapy: A review of empirical studies. *Behavior Modification, 24,* 264–297.

Kleespies, P. M., Deleppo, J. D., Gallagher, P. L., & Niles, B. L. (1999). Managing suicidal emergencies: Recommendations for the practitioner. *Professional Psychology: Research and Practice, 30,* 454–463.

Lambert, M. J., & Bergin, A. E. (1994). The effectiveness of psychotherapy. In A. E. Bergin & S. L. Garfield (Eds.), *Handbook of psychotherapy and behavior change* (4th ed., pp. 143–189). Oxford, UK: Wiley.

Leahy, R. L. (2001). *Overcoming resistance in cognitive therapy.* New York: Guilford Press.

Leahy, R. L. (2003). *Roadblocks in cognitive-behavioral therapy: Transforming challenges into opportunities for change.* New York: Guilford Press.

Maris, R. W. (1992). The relationship of nonfatal suicide attempts to completed suicides. In R. W. Maris & A. L. Berman (Eds.), *Assessment and prediction of suicide* (pp. 362–380). New York: Guilford Press.

Marttunen, M. J., Aro, H. M., & Lönnqvist, J. K. (1993). Precipitant stressors in adolescent suicide. *Journal of the American Academy of Child and Adolescent Psychiatry, 32,* 1178–1183.

McManus, P., Mant, A., Mitchell, P. B., Montgomery, W. S., Marley, J., & Auland, M. E. (2000). Recent trends in the use of antidepressant drugs in Australia, 1990–1998. *Medical Journal of Australia, 173,* 458–461.

Padesky, C. A., & Greenberger, D. (1995). *Clinician's guide to mind over mood.* New York: Guilford Press.

Paykel, E. S., Prusoff, B. A., & Myers, J. K. (1975). Suicide attempts and recent life events: A controlled comparison. *Archives of General Psychiatry, 32,* 327–333.

Persons, J. B. (1989). *Cognitive therapy in practice: A case formulation approach.* New York: Norton.

Rogers, C. R. (1957). The necessary and sufficient conditions of therapeutic personality change. *Journal of Consulting Psychology, 21,* 95–103.

Rudd, M. D., & Joiner, T. (1998). The assessment, management, and treatment of suicidality: Toward clinically informed and balanced standards of care. *Clinical Psychology: Science and Practice, 5,* 135–150.

Sadler, J. Z. (2002). *Descriptions and prescriptions: Values, mental disorders, and the DSMs.* Baltimore, MD: Johns Hopkins University Press.

Shapiro, D. A., & Shapiro, D. (1982). Meta-analysis of comparative therapy outcome studies: A replication and refinement. *Psychological Bulletin, 92,* 581–604.

Smith, M. L., & Glass, G. V. (1977). Meta-analysis of psychotherapy outcome studies. *American Psychologist, 32,* 752–760.

Wierzbicki, M., & Pekarik, G. (1993). A meta-analysis of psychotherapy dropout. *Professional Psychology: Research and Practice, 24,* 190–195.

Wiger, D. E. (1998). *The psychotherapy documentation primer.* Oxford: Wiley.

Wilson, G. T., Fairburn, C. G., & Agras, W. S. (1997). Cognitive behavioral therapy for bulimia nervosa. In D. M. Garner & P. E. Garfinkel (Eds.), *Handbook of treatment for eating disorders* (2nd ed., pp. 67–93). New York: Guilford Press.

INDEX

Absenteeism, 171–173
Academy of Cognitive Therapy, 19
Accomplishment, helping client see, 201–203
Age, questions from client about, 147–149
Agenda, setting for session
  with client, 198–199
  homework and, 181
  importance of, 105–106
American Psychological Association, *Ethical Principles of Psychologists and Code of Conduct*, 26, 27
Anger of client, 190–193
Anxiety
  chattiness and, 189
  downward spiral of, 116–117
  three components of, 115–116
  treatment for, 123–126
Arriving late, 171–173
Assessment
  of additional problems, 44
  for case conceptualization, 16–17
  case example, 56–61
  demographic information and, 40–41, 57
  detail, missing during, 55–56
  for diagnosis, 15–16
  discrepancies between self-report questionnaire and interview, 48
  ending session after, 60–61
  family background and, 44–45
  goals of, 15, 38
  in-session behavior and, 48–49
  Mental Status Exam, 45, 46–47
  mistake, making during, 56
  observation and, 49
  pause or break during, 54–55
  of presenting problem, 41–43, 57–58
  problem list as outcome of, 54, 59–60
  reaction, being mindful of, 36–38
  repeating, to review progress, 202
  self-monitoring, 49–50
  self-report questionnaires, 45, 47–48, 59
  speaking to other professionals, 50–53
  speaking to significant others, 53
  of suicide risk, 140
  See also Interview, clinical; Report writing
Attention, focusing on client, 4, 24–25
Attribution, pattern of, 135–136
Automatic thoughts
  core beliefs and, 11–12
  disputing, 156–159
  logical errors in, 156
  reviewing in therapy session, 155–156
Avoidance behavior
  advantages and disadvantages of, 115–116
  arriving late as, 172–173
  assessment and, 43
  weekly "crisis" and, 106

B

Behavior
  escape, 43
  in-session, 48–49
  See also Avoidance behavior
Behavioral approach, 8–10
Behavior test, 202
Beliefs
  in biological determination, 133–134
  intermediate, 11–12
  irrational, 63
  in need to explore past, 132–133
  See also Core beliefs
Believing rationale, 131
Biological factors, belief difficulties are
    due to, 133–134
Bulimia, treatment of, 154

C

Caller, talking to, 21
Canadian Psychological Association, *Code
    of Ethics for Psychologists*, 26, 27
Case conceptualization
  assessment for, 16–17
  first visit and, 30
  model for cognitive-behavioral, 13
  noncompliance and, 171
  as ongoing process, 78
  origin of mechanism in early life, 69–
    70
  overview of, 4–5, 62–64
  past experience and, 132–133
  precipitants of current problem, 68
  predicted obstacles to treatment, 70–71
  problem list, 54, 59–60, 64
  proposed underlying mechanism, 64–67
  sharing with client, 81, 87–88
  shifts in over time, 164
  stating how proposed mechanism
    produces problem, 68
  treatment plan and, 71–72, 73
  writing notes and, 165
Case example
  assessment, 56–61
  deciding where to start treatment, 77–
    78
  end point for treatment, 196–197
  feedback session, 85–91
  first visit, 34–35
  initial contact, 31–34
  origin of mechanism in early life, 70

overview of treatment, providing, 107–
    110
precipitants of current problem, 68
predicted obstacles to treatment, 70–71
problem list, 64
progress note sample, 168–169
proposed underlying mechanism, 64–67
report, 99–101
session 1, 114–121
session 2, 121–128
session 3, 155–160
session 4, 160–161
session 5, 161–163
sessions 6 to 10, 163–165
stating how proposed mechanism
    produces problem, 68
termination, 210–215
treatment manual, 74
treatment plan, 71–72, 73, 75
Challenges, dealing with
  clinician-related roadblocks, 143–146
  interpersonal issues in therapeutic
    relationship, 146–153
  medication and therapy, 134–137
  socializing clients to CBT, 130–134
  staying positive, 195
  suicidal client, 137–138
  in supervisory relationship, 224–232
  See also Noncompliance
Change
  attributions for, 135–136
  fear of, 183–184
Choosing supervisor, 219–220
Classical conditioning, 8–9
Cognitive approach, 8, 10–12
Cognitive-behavioral therapy (CBT)
  commonly asked questions about, 91–
    97
  determining when inappropriate, 84–85
  explaining to client, 82–84
  See also Theoretical basis of CBT
Cognitive restructuring
  continuing, 160–161, 163–165
  explaining to client, 125
  introducing, 155–160
  overview of, 12–14
Collaboration with client
  agenda, setting, 105–106
  case conceptualization and, 5
  See also Therapeutic alliance
Collaborative empiricism, stance of, 83–
    84, 92

Communication with other professionals, 50–53, 165–167
Conditioned stimulus and response, 8–9
Confidentiality
    discussing, 29–30, 31
    mode of transmission of information and, 50
    office environment and, 24
Connection between past experience and current beliefs and behavior, 132–133
Consent
    information to cover in, 28–29, 31
    obtaining, 27–28, 31, 89–91
Consultation with colleagues, 138
Coordination of treatment with prescribing physician, 134–135, 137
Core beliefs
    applying cognitive model to, 69
    description of, 11–12
    family background and, 44–45
    reasoning inductively toward, 63–64
Cost–benefit analysis, helping client conduct, 175–176
Crying in front of client, 38

D

Demographic information, 40–41, 57
Desire, suicidal, 141–142
Diagnosis
    assessment for, 15–16
    reviewing with client, 81
    suicide risk and, 141
Diagnostic and Statistical Manual of Mental Disorders, 4th edition, text revision, 15
Difficulties
    asking client about, 21
    being mindful of potential, 5–6
    overt, 62–63
    in therapeutic alliance, 146–153
    See also Challenges, dealing with; Normalizing difficulties
Disagreement with supervisor, 229
Discontinuing medication, 136–137
Discounting of approach by client, 131–132
Disputing negative thoughts, 156–159
Diversionary tactics of client, 176–180

Documentation
    content of, 166–167
    importance of, 165–166
    progress note sample, 168–169
    suicide assessment and, 137–138
    See also Report writing

E

Early experience, belief in need to explore, 132–133
Early termination
    by client, 208–209
    by clinician, 207–208
    due to success, 206–207
Effectiveness of CBT, 92–94
Emotions and automatic thoughts, 155–156
Empathy, 4
Encouraging homework compliance, 181–183
Ending therapy session with summary, 119–120
End point for treatment, 196–197
Ensuring competent care with supervision, 218
Escape behaviors, 43
Ethical dilemma, resolving, 229
Evaluation
    by supervisor, 227–228
    of supervisor, 232
Expectations
    early termination and, 208
    establishing for future, 204–205
Experience, questions from client about, 147–149
Exposures
    explaining to client, 124–125
    first, 161–163
    hierarchy for, development of, 127–128
    in vivo, 14–15, 135
    medication and, 135
    planning, 160–161
Extending treatment, 209–210

F

Family background, 44–45
Fear
    of change, 183–184
    of evaluation by supervisor, 227–228
    of incompetence, 7

Fear (continued)
of judgment by clinician, 183, 186
of sharing information, 188
of therapy, dealing with, 174–176
Fee, setting and explaining policies related
to, 23
Feedback from client, permitting and
encouraging, 121
Feedback to client
on case conceptualization, 81, 87–88
guidelines for, 79, 80
on problem list and diagnosis, 80–81,
86–87
on strengths, 79–80, 85–86
on treatment options, 82–85, 88–89,
91
"Firing" client, 207–208
First treatment session
case example, 114–121
introductions, reviews, and check-ins,
106–107
overview of treatment, providing, 107–
110
preparing for, 104
psychoeducational component of, 110–
113
tips for, 129
First visit
advance mailing, asking permission to
send, 22–23
case conceptualization and, 30
case example, 34–35
confidentiality, discussing, 29–30
consent, obtaining, 27–29, 31
fee, setting, 23
giving overview of, 27, 34–35
greeting client, 25
introduction and permission to record,
obtaining, 25–27
setting up, 22, 34
social graces and, 25
Flirting by client, 152–153
Fortune-telling error, 156

G

Generalization, 9
Genuineness, 4
Gift from client, 150–151
Goals
setting prior to termination, 203–204
of supervision, 216–217

Greeting client, 25
Group supervision, 221–222
Guidance, heavy-handed, by supervisor,
225

H

Hierarchy
development of, 127–128
review of, 202–203
History
of suicide attempt, 141
of treatment, 43, 94–96
Homework
client design of, 198
explaining to client, 125–126
introducing, 120–121
resistance to, 180–183
reviewing, 122
use of in CBT, 128–129
Hopelessness and suicide risk, 141

I

"If-then" statements, 63
Impulsivity and suicide risk, 141
Inappropriate behavior by supervisor,
230–232
Incompetence, fears of, 7
Individual supervision, 221–222
Informed decision about treatment,
helping client make, 82–84
Initial contact by phone
case example, 31–34
making recommendations, 21–22, 33–34
responding to, 20–21
In-session work, resistance to, 173–176
Intermediate beliefs, 11–12
Interview, clinical
discrepancies between self-report
questionnaire and, 48
repeating, to review progress, 202
semistructured, 16, 39–40, 58–59
unstructured, 40–45
Introductions, 25, 26, 106
Invitation from client to social event,
151–152
In vivo exposure
description of, 14–15
medication and, 135
Irrational beliefs, 63
Irritability in client, 190–193

J

Judgment, fear of
  by clinician, 183, 186
  by supervisor, 227–228

L

Labeling, 156
Language of client, using, 42
Lapses, planning for, 204–206
Lateness of client, 171–173
Learning
  observing and, 16, 18–19
  practice and, 7
Learning theory, 14
Life events, stressful, 140
Live observation, 224

M

Manuals, treatment, 73–74, 75
Medication
  attributions for change and, 135–136
  coordination of treatment with
    prescribing physician, 134–135,
    137
  discontinuing, 136–137
  negative impact on CBT by, 135
  questions or concerns about, 96–97, 135
Membership in professional organizations,
  19
Mental filter, 156
Mental Status Exam, 45, 46–47
Mentoring, 218
Mind-reading error, 156
Missing session, 171–173
Model for disorder, drawing diagram of,
  112
Moral dilemma, resolving, 229

N

Name of client, using, 25
Noncompliance
  difficulty with therapeutic relationship
    and, 184–185
  diversionary tactics, 176–180
  with homework, 180–183
  missing sessions or arriving late, 171–173
  overview of, 170–171
  reluctance to open up, 185–188
  resistance to in-session work, 173–176

Normalizing difficulties
  during assessment, 37
  during first contact, 21
  psychoeducation and, 111
  as relapse prevention, 205
  suicidal thoughts, 139

O

Observation
  as assessment option, 49
  of experienced clinician, 16, 18–19
  supervision and, 224
Open up, reluctance to, 185–188
Operant conditioning, 9–10
Orientations, conflicting, between
    clinician and supervisor, 225–
    227
Over-compliance by client, 193–195

P

Pace of therapy, 131
Panic attack, treatment of, 154
Past, belief in need to explore, 132–133
Perception in cognitive model, 10–11
Permission form, 50, 53
Personal questions from client, dealing
    with, 146–150
Persuasion, harm in using, 83–84
Phobia
  social, 33
  in vivo exposure and, 14–15
Physician, prescribing, coordination of
    treatment with, 134–135, 137
Plan for suicide, assessing, 141
Positive, staying, 195
Practice and learning, 7
Praising client, 201
Predisposing factors for suicide, 139
Preparation
  adequate, 1–2, 6–7
  emotional, 7–8
  for new client, 23–24, 104
  observing and, 16, 18–19
  for psychoeducation component of
    treatment, 113
  reading and, 17–18
Presenting problem
  assessment of, 41–43
  case example, 57–58
  reviewing, 107

Problem list
    deciding where to start with, 74, 76–78
    as outcome of assessment, 54, 59–60,
        64
    reviewing with client, 80–81, 86–87
Process
    case conceptualization, 4–5
    difficulties, being mindful of potential,
        5–6
    overview of, 2–3
    therapeutic alliance, establishing and
        maintaining, 3–4
Professional organizations, membership
    in, 19
Progress, reviewing with client, 201–203
Progress notes. *See* Documentation
Progress note sample, 168–169
Protective factors and suicide risk, 142
Psychoeducation component of treatment
    content of, 111–112
    as discussion rather than lecture, 112–
        113
    family background, early life, and,
        122–123
    fear and, 174
    purpose of, 110–111
    tip sheet for, 113, 114

Q

Questionnaires, self-report, 45, 47–48, 59,
    203
Questions
    permitting and encouraging, 121
    personal, from client, dealing with,
        146–150
    Socratic, 83–84, 110

R

Rapport, establishing
    interview and, 39–40
    psychoeducation component of
        treatment and, 110
    between supervisor and trainee, 228–
        232
    See also Therapeutic alliance,
        establishing and maintaining
Rational response, 159
Reactions to client
    during assessment, 36–38
    homework and, 183

negative, 145–146
    suicide assessment and, 138–139
Recordkeeping. *See* Documentation
Referral source, speaking to, 51–52
Reinforcement, 9–10, 181
Relapse, planning for, 204–206
Reluctance to open up, 185–188
Report writing
    assessment results section, 102
    background information section, 101–
        102
    behavioral observations section, 101
    case example, 99–101
    elements to include, 103
    evaluation procedures section, 98, 101
    general information section, 98
    general rules for, 97–98
    impressions and interpretations section,
        102
    recommendations section, 103
    referral question section, 98
    See also Documentation
Resistance. *See* Noncompliance
Resources
    anxiety disorders, 234–235
    bipolar disorder, 235
    case conceptualization, 17
    children, 235–236
    clinical applications, 234, 239–240
    core techniques, 17
    depression and suicide, 236
    eating disorders, 236–237
    group therapy, 237
    journals, 241–242
    marriage and family problems, 237
    medical problems, 237
    obsessive–compulsive disorder, 237
    older adults, 238
    personality disorders, 238
    resistance, 238
    schizophrenia, 238–239
    substance abuse, 238
    theoretical basis of CBT, 18
    theory and research, 233–234
    websites, 242
Risk factors for suicide, 140–142
Roadblocks, clinician-related
    difficulties in therapeutic relationship,
        144–146
    issues affecting approach to case, 143–
        144
Roles of supervisor, 217–218

S

Safety contract with suicidal client, 142–143
Second treatment session
    case example, 121–128
    tips for, 129
Self-focus of beginning clinician, 4, 24–25
Self-handicapping strategy, 172
Self-monitoring, 49–50, 202
Self-report method of supervision, 222–223
Self-report questionnaires, 45, 47–48, 59
Session
    agenda, setting for, 105–106, 181, 198–199
    behavior during, 48–49
    ending after assessment, 60–61
    ending with summary, 119–120
    missing or arriving late to, 171–173
    second, 121–129
    taping, 26–27, 223–224
    See also First treatment session
Sexual harassment by supervisor, 230–232
Significant others, speaking to, 53
Skills, process
    case conceptualization, 4–5
    therapeutic alliance, establishing and maintaining, 3–4
Socializing clients to CBT
    belief in biological determination, 133–134
    belief in exploration of early experience, 132–133
    difficulty with approach, 131–132
    pace of therapy, 131
Social phobia, 33
Social support, 142
Socratic questioning, 83–84, 110
Speaking to other professionals, 50–53, 165–167
Strengths, reviewing with client, 79–80, 85–86
Stressors
    presenting problem and, 176–180
    suicide risk and, 140
Success at homework, 182–183
Successful outcome, definition of, 7–8
Suicidal client, working with
    assessment questions for, 140
    consultation and, 138
    documentation and, 137–138

emotional reaction to threat, 138–139
    factors, knowing, 139
    legalities of, 137
    predisposing factors, 139
    protective factors, 142
    risk factors, 140–142
    supervision when, 138
    treating, 142–143
Supervision
    anxiety and, 6
    case conceptualization and, 17
    choosing supervisor, 219–220
    dealing with roadblocks in relationship, 224–232
    defining relationship, 220
    difficulties in way cases are understood and treated, 225–227
    disagreement on moral or ethical issues, 229
    evaluation of, 232
    fear of evaluation, 227–228
    goals of, 216–217
    individual versus group, 221–222
    lack of time for, 228–229
    providing name of supervisor to client, 26
    roles of, 217–218
    sexual harassment and, 230–232
    sharing work, 222–224
    suicidal client, working with, 138
    therapist role compared to, 229–230
    trainee role in, 218–219
Symptoms
    case conceptualization and, 5
    cause of, 4
    underreporting or denial of, 48

T

Take-home messages, 119–120, 128
Talkativeness of client, 188–190
Taping sessions
    obtaining permission for, 26–27
    for supervision, 223–224
Teaching client to be own clinician, 197–201
Tearing up in front of client, 38
Techniques
    resources on, 17
    Socratic questioning, 83–84, 110
    See also Cognitive restructuring; Exposures

Termination
  case example, 210–215
  early, 206–209
  end point for treatment, keeping in
    mind, 196–197
  expectations, establishing for future,
    204–205
  goals, setting, 203–204
  last few sessions of therapy, 201–206
  progress, reviewing, 201–203
  relapse, planning for, 204–206
  teaching client to be own clinician,
    197–201
Theoretical basis of CBT
  behavioral approach, 8–10
  cognitive approach, 10–12
  cognitive-behavioral integration, 12–15
  overview of, 8
  resources on, 18
Therapeutic alliance
  angry, irritable client and, 190–193
  clinician difficulties in, 144–146
  difficult interpersonal situations and,
    146–153
  establishing and maintaining, 3–4
  noncompliance and, 171
  over-compliance and, 193–195
  reluctance to open up and, 185–188
  talking too much and, 188–190
  See also Rapport, establishing
Thinking, dysfunctional, 10–11
Time, lack of
  as excuse for not doing homework,
    182
  by supervisor, 228–229
Time-limited nature of CBT, 84, 94
Tip sheet, 113, 114
Tone of therapy, controlling, 191

Trainee role in supervision, 218–219
Training and supervision, 217–218
Training programs, 1–2
Treatment
  for clinician, 144
  end point for, 196–197
  extending, 209–210
  informed decision about, helping client
    make, 82–84
  by supervisor of trainee, 229–230
  See also Psychoeducation component of
    treatment
Treatment history
  assessment and, 43
  failure of CBT in past, 94–96
Treatment plan
  case conceptualization and, 71–72, 73
  case example, 75
  consent, obtaining for, 89–91
  deciding where to start in, 74, 76–78
  end point for, 196–197
  reviewing with client, 82–85, 88–89
  shifts in over time, 164
  therapy manuals and, 73–74, 75

U

Unconditional positive regard, 4
Unconditioned stimulus and response, 8–9
Underlying psychological mechanisms, 63,
  64–67
Understanding purpose of techniques, 131

W

Waiting room, 25
Warmth, nonpossessive, 4
World Rounds Videotapes, 18–19